SPRINGHOUSE

N O T E S™

CRITICAL CARE AND EMERGENCY NURSING

Sandra Smith Huddleston, RN, MSN, CCRN

Ms. Huddleston, coauthor of this book, is an Assistant Professor of Nursing at Berea College, Berea, Ky. She earned her BSN from Eastern Kentucky University, Richmond, and received her MSN from the University of Kentucky, Lexington. Ms. Huddleston is a member of the American Association of Critical-Care Nurses and Sigma Theta Tau and is listed in *Who's Who in American Nursing*.

Sondra G. Ferguson, RN, MSN, CS

Ms. Ferguson, coauthor of this book, is a Clinical Nurse Specialist for Critical Care at the Veterans Administration Medical,Center in Lexington, Ky. She received her BSN and MSN from the University of Kentucky, Lexington. Ms. Ferguson is a member of the American Association of Critical-Care Nurses, the American Nurses' Association, the Kentucky Nurses' Association, Sigma Theta Tau, and the Nurses Organization of the Veterans Administration.

Michaelene P. Mirr, RN, PhD, CCRN

Dr. Mirr, reviewer of this book, is an Associate Professor of Nursing at the University of Wisconsin, Eau Claire. She received her BSN from the University of Wisconsin, Eau Claire; her MSN from the University of Wisconsin, Madison; and her PhD from the University of Minnesota. Dr. Mirr is a member of the American Association of Critical-Care Nurses, American Association of Neuroscience Nurses, American Nurses' Association, American Association for the History of Nursing, and the Midwest Nursing Research Society.

Springhouse Corporation
Springhouse, Pennsylvania

Staff

Executive Director, Editorial
Stanley Loeb

Executive Director, Creative Services
Jean Robinson

Director of Trade and Textbooks
Minnie B. Rose, RN, BSN, MEd

Art Director
John Hubbard

Acquisitions Editor
Donna L. Hilton, RN, BSN, CEN

Consultant
Maryann Foley, RN, BSN

Editorial Manager
Kevin Law

Editor
David Moreau

Copy Editors
Keith de Pinho, Nancy Papsin, Doris Weinstock

Designers
Stephanie Peters (associate art director),
Julie Carleton Barlow

Art Production
Robert Perry (manager), Anna Brindisi, Donald
Knauss, Catherine Mace, Robert Wieder

Typography
David Kosten (manager), Diane Paluba (assistant
manager), Joyce Rossi Biletz, Brenda C. Mayer,
Robin Rantz, Brent Rinedoller, Valerie L.
Rosenberger

Manufacturing
Deborah Meiris (manager), T.A. Landis, Jennifer
Suter

Production Coordination
Aline S. Miller (manager), Laura L. Williams

Library of Congress Cataloging-in-Publication Data

Huddleston, Sandra Smith.
  Critical care and emergency nursing/Sandra
  Smith Huddleston, Sondra G. Ferguson.
    p. cm. — (Springhouse notes)
  Includes bibliographical references.
  1. Intensive care nursing. 2. Emergency
  nursing. I. Ferguson, Sondra
  G. II. Title. III. Series.
  [DNLM: 1. Critical Care—nurses'
  instruction. 2. Emergencies—nurses'
  instruction. WY 154 H884c]
RT120.I5H83 1990
610.73'61—dc20
DNLM/DLC   89-21605
ISBN 0-87434-227-9   CIP

Contents

How to Use Springhouse Notes

Today, more than ever, nursing students face enormous time pressures. Nursing education has become more sophisticated, increasing the difficulties students have with studying efficiently and keeping pace.

The need for a comprehensive, well-designed series of study aids is great, which is why we've produced Springhouse Notes...to meet that need. Springhouse Notes provide essential course material in outline form, enabling the nursing student to study more effectively, improve understanding, achieve higher test scores, and get better grades.

Key features appear throughout each book, making the information more accessible and easier to remember.
- **Learning Objectives.** These objectives precede each section in the book to help the student evaluate knowledge before and after study.
- **Key Points.** Highlighted in color throughout the book, these points provide a way to quickly review critical information. Key points may include:
—a cardinal sign or symptom of a disorder
—the most current or popular theory about a topic
—a distinguishing characteristic of a disorder
—the most important step of a process
—a critical assessment component
—a crucial nursing intervention
—the most widely used or successful therapy or treatment.
- **Points to Remember.** This information, found at the end of each section, summarizes the section in capsule form.
- **Glossary.** Difficult, frequently used, or sometimes misunderstood terms are defined for the student at the end of each section.

Remember: Springhouse Notes are learning tools designed to *help* you. They are not intended for use as a primary information source. They should never substitute for class attendance, text reading, or classroom note-taking.

This book, *Critical Care and Emergency Nursing,* begins with perspectives, physiologic concepts, and psychosocial aspects of critical care and emergency nursing. It then outlines important aspects of nutritional support, infection control, emergency life support, mechanical ventilation, hemodynamic monitoring, intracranial pressure monitoring, continuous cardiac monitoring, and dysrhythmias. Subsequent sections, organized by body system, begin with general information about the body system and then present subsections on specific diseases and disorders. Each subsection includes general information, causes, assessment findings, diagnostic test findings, and patient care management. The book concludes with sections on multisystemic disorders and trauma.

Perspectives on Critical Care and Emergency Nursing

Learning Objectives

After studying this section, the reader should be able to:

- Identify general principles related to patients requiring critical care and emergency nursing.

- Differentiate among the independent, dependent, and interdependent interventions of critical care and emergency nurses.

- Describe the concept of triage in emergency nursing.

- Discuss the roles and functions of critical care and emergency nurses.

- Name legal and ethical issues that can affect critical care or emergency nursing.

I. Perspectives on Critical Care and Emergency Nursing

A. Introduction

1. Critical care and emergency nursing are separate specialties within the scope of nursing practice, with the common goal of restoring physiologic or psychological stability to the severely ill patient
2. Because these two nursing specialties encompass all areas of practice, critical care and emergency nurses must have knowledge and skill beyond those of the nurse generalist
   a. Both have a core body of knowledge of principles and techniques that apply to medicine, surgery, pediatrics, obstetrics, and psychiatry
   b. Both have core concepts that are essential components of adequate assessment and that form the cornerstone of appropriate therapy in critical care and emergency areas
   c. Both use the nursing process as a framework for practice
3. Critical care and emergency nursing encompass independent, dependent, and interdependent interventions
   a. *Independent* nursing interventions are unique to nursing and include management of the environment, teaching, counseling, and initiating referrals
   b. *Dependent* nursing interventions are prescribed by medicine
   c. *Interdependent* nursing interventions are determined by multidisciplinary collaboration
4. Critical care and emergency nurses are often responsible for making life-and-death decisions, placing them at a high legal risk
   a. Priorities must be determined quickly, based on sound knowledge and judgment
   b. Triage decisions must be made to expedite care
5. Critical care and emergency nurses are at high risk of injury or illness from possible exposure to infections, such as hepatitis, acquired immunodeficiency syndrome (AIDS), or other communicable diseases

B. Critical care nursing

1. General information
   a. Critical care nursing deals with human responses to life-threatening problems and includes the critically ill patient, the critical care nurse, and the critical care environment
   b. Care is provided to patients of all ages with alterations in physical or emotional health
   c. The critically ill patient is at high risk for developing life-threatening problems and requires constant, intensive, multidisciplinary assessment and intervention to restore stability, prevent complications, and achieve and maintain optimal responses
   d. The critical care nurse coordinates interventions aimed at resolving life-threatening problems

2. Historical development
    a. Critical care began as a component of recovery rooms before expanding into coronary care units in the 1960s
    b. The American Association of Critical-Care Nurses (AACN) was organized in 1969
    c. A competency-based examination was developed in 1975 to provide certification in critical care nursing (CCRN); certification is valid for 3 years
    d. The AACN developed Standards for Nursing Care of the Critically Ill in 1981 to explain the role of the critical care nurse in ensuring quality care for critically ill patients and their families
3. Critical care environment
    a. Units may be specifically designated as medical, surgical, coronary, pediatric, neonatal, recovery, or postanesthesia or may encompass other areas in some institutions
    b. Adequate resources (emergency equipment, supplies, and support systems) are necessary for safe care
    c. A management and administrative structure is required to ensure effective care through all phases of the patient's hospital stay, from emergency department to discharge
    d. Legal, regulatory, social, economic, and political trends must be monitored to promote the early recognition of problems and a timely response
    e. Specialized electronic technology and techniques are used to monitor patient status continuously; these may create safety hazards for patients, such as possible exposure to electric shock
4. Roles of the critical care nurse
    a. Care provider: provides comprehensive—and at times highly technical—direct care to the patient and family in response to life-threatening health problems
    b. Educator: provides patient and family with education based on their learning needs and the severity of the situation and allows the patient to assume more responsibility for meeting health care needs as health condition stabilizes or improves
    c. Manager: coordinates the care delivered by various health care workers to achieve the specific goal of providing optimal nursing care to critically ill patients
    d. Advocate: protects the patient's rights
5. Functions of the critical care nurse
    a. Assesses and implements treatment for patient responses to life-threatening health problems
    b. Provides direct measures to resuscitate, if necessary
    c. Uses independent, dependent, and interdependent interventions to restore stability, prevent complications, and achieve and maintain optimal patient responses
    d. Provides health education to the patient and family

    e. Supervises patient care and ancillary personnel

    f. Supports patient adaptation, restores health, and preserves the patient's rights, including the right to refuse treatment

  6. Legal issues affecting the delivery of critical care nursing

    a. Negligence

    b. Malpractice

    c. Informed consent

    d. Implied consent

  7. Ethical issues affecting the delivery of critical care nursing

    a. Ethnic and religious doctrines that limit treatment options

    b. Allocation of resources that may limit admissions or promote premature discharges

    c. Use of critical care beds for terminally ill patients

    d. Discontinuation of resuscitation or life-support measures

    e. Do-not-resuscitate (DNR) orders

    f. Living wills

C. Emergency nursing

  1. General information

    a. Emergency nursing deals with human responses to any trauma or sudden illness that requires immediate intervention to prevent imminent severe damage or death

    b. Care is provided in any setting to individuals of all ages with actual or perceived alterations in physical or emotional health

    c. Initially, patients may not have a medical diagnosis

    d. Care is *episodic* when patients return frequently, *primary* when it is the only option for health care, or *acute* when patients need immediate and additional interventions

  2. Historical development

    a. Florence Nightingale was the first emergency nurse, providing care to the wounded in the Crimean War in 1854

    b. The Emergency Department Nurses Association (EDNA) was organized in 1970

    c. A competency-based examination, first administered in 1980, provides Certification in Emergency Nursing (CEN); certification is valid for 4 years

    d. EDNA developed Standards of Emergency Nursing Practice, published in 1983, to be used as guidelines for excellence and outcome criteria against which performance is measured and evaluated

    e. EDNA changed its name to the Emergency Nurses Association (ENA) in 1985 to encompass a practice setting larger than the emergency room

  3. Emergency care environment

    a. Prehospital care by emergency medical services (EMS), emergency medical technicians (EMTs), and paramedics provides initial stabilization and transport of patients; personnel communicate with the emergency department during patient transport

  b. The national emergency telephone number 911 is the result of an effort
     to improve access to EMS
  c. The concept of the emergency room has expanded to that of the
     emergency department, which provides various levels of care
  d. Specialized electronic technology and techniques are used to monitor
     patient status continuously; these may pose safety hazards to patients,
     such as possible exposure to electric shock
4. Triage
  a. Triage classifies emergency patients for assessment and treatment
     priorities
  b. Triage decisions require gathering objective and subjective data rapidly
     and effectively to determine the type of priority situation present
  c. *Emergent situations* are potentially life-threatening; they include such
     conditions as respiratory distress or arrest, cardiac arrest, severe chest
     pain, seizures, hemorrhage, severe trauma resulting in open chest or
     abdominal wounds, shock, poisonings, drug overdoses, temperatures over
     105° F. (40.5° C.), emergency childbirth, or delivery complications
  d. *Urgent situations* are serious but not life-threatening if treatment is
     delayed briefly; they include such conditions as chest pain without
     respiratory distress, major fractures, burns, decreased level of
     consciousness, back injuries, nausea or vomiting, severe abdominal pain,
     temperature between 102° F. (38.9° C.) and 105° F., bleeding from any
     orifice, acute panic, or anxiety
  e. *Nonemergency situations* are not acute and are considered minor to
     moderately severe; they include such conditions as chronic backache or
     other complaints, moderate headache, minor burns, fractures, sprains,
     upper respiratory or urinary infections, or instances in which a patient is
     dead on arrival
5. Roles of the emergency nurse
  a. Care provider: provides comprehensive direct care to the patient and
     family
  b. Educator: provides patient and family with education based on their
     learning needs and the severity of the situation and allows the patient to
     assume more responsibility for meeting health care needs
  c. Manager: coordinates activities of others in the multidisciplinary team to
     achieve the specific goal of providing emergency care
  d. Advocate: ensures protection of the patient's rights
6. Functions of the emergency nurse
  a. Uses triage to determine priorities based on assessment and anticipation
     of the patient's needs
  b. Provides direct measures to resuscitate, if necessary
  c. Provides preliminary care before the patient is transferred to the primary
     care area
  d. Provides health education to the patient and family
  e. Supervises patient care and ancillary personnel
  f. Provides support and protection for the patient and family

7. Legal issues affecting the delivery of emergency nursing
   a. Negligence
   b. Malpractice
   c. Good Samaritan Laws (these statutes may protect private citizens but usually do not apply to emergency personnel on duty or in normal emergency situations)
   d. Informed consent
   e. Implied consent
   f. Duty to report suspected crimes to the police
   g. Duty to gather evidence in criminal investigations
8. Ethical issues affecting the delivery of emergency nursing
   a. Ethnic and religious doctrines that limit treatment options
   b. Allocation of emergency care resources that may limit admissions or promote premature discharges
   c. Decisions to stop resuscitation efforts or to resuscitate terminal cases
   d. Living wills

Points to Remember

Critical care and emergency nursing are two separate specialties within the scope of nursing practice that have a common goal of restoring physiologic or psychological stability to a critically ill patient.

Triage decisions require gathering objective and subjective data rapidly and effectively.

Critical care and emergency nursing are high-risk occupations from a legal standpoint.

Ethical dilemmas affect the delivery of care for critically ill and emergency patients.

Glossary

DNR (do not resuscitate)—written order not to initiate resuscitative measures based on the patient's and family's request or the patient's clinical condition

Informed consent—permission for treatment given by the patient after he has received sufficient information to make a decision about his health care

Malpractice—act of omission or commission in which the nurse fails to conform to an identified standard of practice and causes the patient harm; it may include such acts as failing to observe or report changes in the patient's condition, failing to obtain informed consent, or administering the wrong drug to a patient

Triage—method of decision making used by emergency nurses to determine which patients should be treated first and where treatment should take place

Physiologic Concepts Essential to Critical Care and Emergency Nursing

Learning Objectives

After studying this section, the reader should be able to:

• Identify the core concepts essential to critical care and emergency nursing.

• Describe the regulatory mechanism used to maintain homeostasis for each concept.

• Discuss the application of each concept to critical care and emergency nursing.

II. Physiologic Concepts Essential to Critical Care and Emergency Nursing

A. Introduction
1. Core concepts imply that common principles relate to patients in both critical care and emergency areas
2. These concepts are generalized ideas and standard elements that provide a sensible approach to mastering the principles and skills of critical care and emergency nursing
3. Core concepts are essential for rapid patient assessment and provide the foundation for nursing activities and interventions in the emergency department and critical care areas
4. Core concepts in this section include:
   a. Acid-base balance
   b. Fluid and electrolyte balance
   c. Tissue perfusion
   d. Gas exchange
5. These concepts often blend and overlap, an imbalance in one causing an imbalance in one or more of the others

B. Acid-base balance
1. General information
   a. The normal ratio of acid to base is 1:20, representing one part acid, such as carbon dioxide (CO_2), to 20 parts base, such as bicarbonate ($HCO_3{}^-$)
   b. Metabolic processes must maintain a steady balance of acids and bases to ensure optimum cellular functioning
   c. An acid is any substance that can donate or give up hydrogen ions (H^+)
   d. A base is any substance that can accept H^+
   e. Acid-base balance is measured by arterial blood gas (ABG) analysis

NORMAL A.B.G. VALUES	
pH	7.35 to 7.45
$PaCO_2$	35 to 45 mm Hg
HCO_3-	22 to 26 mEq/liter
PaO_2	80 to 100 mm Hg
O_2 Sat	95% to 100%
Base excess	-2.5 to $+2.5$

   f. Arterial blood pH is an indirect measurement of hydrogen ion concentration
   g. Arterial blood carbon dioxide ($PaCO_2$) measures the partial pressure of carbon dioxide in arterial blood. It reflects alveolar ventilation and is the respiratory component of acid-base balance
   h. Arterial blood bicarbonate (HCO_3-) reflects the metabolic component of acid-base balance

      i. Arterial blood oxygen (PaO_2) measures the partial pressure of oxygen in arterial blood and reflects the adequacy of oxygenation

      j. Arterial blood oxygen saturation measures the percentage of hemoglobin saturated with oxygen

      k. Arterial blood base excess reflects the amount of buffering present

      l. Body temperature and oxygen content of inspired air must be determined for accurate ABG analysis

  2. Regulation

      a. Acids are continuously liberated as metabolic by-products

      b. Body buffer systems prevent large changes in pH by chemically combining acids with other ions

      c. The respiratory system is responsible for regulating the body's CO_2 level; the renal system is responsible for regulating the body's HCO_3^- level

      d. Compensation occurs as a response by the system not primarily affected to minimize changes in pH or to return pH to near normal

      e. Respiratory imbalances result in metabolic compensation by the kidneys, which may take several days

      f. Metabolic imbalances result in respiratory compensation by the lungs, which begins in minutes

      g. Correction of acid-base imbalances to return the pH to normal depends on a physiologic or therapeutic response by the system primarily affected

  3. Application to critical care and emergency nursing

      a. Patients admitted to critical care or emergency areas typically suffer from conditions that alter acid-base balance

      b. Patients with acid-base imbalances experience various changes that disrupt overall body functioning

      c. Knowledge of acid-base balance, compensation, and correction is crucial to promote optimum body functioning

      d. Knowledge of normal and abnormal ABG values indicating acid-base balance or imbalance is essential for effective patient care management

      e. Patient care management is aimed at restoring and maintaining acid-base balance

C. Fluid and electrolyte balance

  1. General information

      a. Fluid and electrolyte balance describes the body's normal ratio of water to electrolytes within body fluids

      b. Water in the body carries nutrients and waste material and is expressed as a percentage of body weight

      c. The amount of water in the body is related to age, sex, and body fat; in adults, water content is 60% of body weight in the average male and 50% in the average female; the elderly have a lower percentage of body water, and children have a greater percentage

      d. Body water is distributed between two major fluid compartments: extracellular and intracellular

    e. *Extracellular fluid* (ECF) constitutes one-third of total body water and is found in the blood vessels as plasma and between the cells as interstitial fluid

    f. *Intracellular fluid* (ICF) constitutes two-thirds of total body water and is found within the cell

    g. Electrolytes are positively or negatively charged substances that unite in various combinations in body fluids and differ in concentration in ECF and ICF

    h. Major ECF electrolytes include sodium (Na^+, the principal cation), chloride (Cl^-), and bicarbonate (HCO_3^-)

    i. Major ICF electrolytes include potassium (K^+), magnesium (Mg^{++}), phosphates, and proteins

    j. Fluid (water and electrolytes) moves between compartments; fluid movement is determined by the permeability of the membrane separating the fluid compartments, fluid osmolality, ECF concentration of Na^+, the crystalloid and colloidal osmostic pressure, and capillary hydrostatic pressure

    k. Mechanisms by which water and electrolytes move between fluid compartments include diffusion, osmosis, and active transport (sodium-potassium pump)

2. Regulation

    a. Compensatory mechanisms maintain fluid and electrolyte levels within normal range

    b. For homeostasis to occur, fluid intake must equal fluid output; average daily fluid intake is approximately 2,600 ml; average daily fluid output is 2,600 ml, which includes water lost as urine, in stool, and through the lungs and skin

    c. Specific organs and glands also help to regulate fluid and electrolyte balance

    d. Kidneys perform major regulatory functions, including retention and excretion of fluids and select electrolytes, regulation of pH and excretion of metabolic waste and toxic substances, and secretion of renin as a response to decreased blood pressure or ECF volume

    e. Through its pumping action, the heart maintains the kidneys' perfusion pressure to regulate water and electrolyte balance

    f. The lungs maintain acid-base balance and contribute to insensible water loss; renin interacts with angiotensinogen in the liver to form angiotensin I, which converts to angiotensin II, a potent vasopressor, in the lungs

    g. The adrenal glands secrete aldosterone, which alters the fluid balance. Increased aldosterone secretion retains Na^+, increasing water retention and K^+ loss; decreased aldosterone secretion causes Na^+ and water loss and K^+ retention; angiotensin II stimulates the secretion and production of aldosterone

    h. The hypothalamus responds to increased serum osmolality, which stimulates the thirst center and the need for water ingestion; it also produces antidiuretic hormone (ADH)

      i. The posterior pituitary gland secretes ADH, causing fluid retention. The primary stimulus for secretion is serum osmolality; the secondary stimulus is a severe ECF deficit

      j. The parathyroid glands regulate calcium and phosphate by secreting parathyroid hormone, which affects bone resorption and calcium absorption and reabsorption

  3. Application to critical care and emergency nursing

    a. Healthy individuals can cope with changes in fluid and electrolyte composition

    b. Patients admitted to critical care or emergency areas typically suffer from conditions that alter their fluid and electrolyte balance or restrict their ability to eat and drink to maintain an equilibrium in fluids and electrolytes

    c. Patients experience various changes that disrupt both physiologic and psychological integrity because of fluid and electrolye imbalances

    d. Patient care management is aimed at restoring and maintaining fluid and electrolyte balance

D. Tissue perfusion

  1. General information

    a. Tissue perfusion is the process by which blood flow to the cells provides nutrients necessary for proper cellular functioning

    b. Adequate tissue perfusion is essential to adequate cellular functioning and homeostasis

    c. Adequate tissue perfusion provides cells with the oxygen necessary for metabolic processes and waste removal

    d. Decreased tissue perfusion decreases oxygen to the cells (tissue hypoxia), leading to anaerobic metabolism and accumulation of waste products in the cells

    e. These processes further result in lactic acidosis and shock

  2. Regulation

    a. Compensatory mechanisms are activated by inadequate tissue perfusion

    b. Baroreceptors in the carotid and aortic arch stimulate the vasomotor center in the medulla

    c. The sympathetic nervous system releases epinephrine and norepinephrine

    d. Blood is shunted to vital organs (the heart and brain) and away from organs that tolerate ischemia (skin, skeletal muscles, and fat)

    e. The respiratory rate increases to improve oxygenation

    f. The renin-angiotensin-aldosterone system is activated to increase water retention

    g. The posterior pituitary gland secretes ADH or vasopressin, a potent vasoconstrictor, to increase water retention

  3. Application to critical care and emergency nursing

    a. Patients admitted to critical care or emergency areas typically suffer from conditions that adversely affect tissue perfusion

b. As abnormal tissue perfusion occurs, shock develops, leading to alterations in tissue metabolism and to death of tissue cells

c. Accurate assessment of tissue perfusion and prompt intervention can improve the patient's chances for survival

E. Gas exchange

1. General information

a. Gas exchange describes two processes: the movement of oxygen (O_2) from the alveoli to the bloodstream, where it is bound to hemoglobin and transported to the cells; and the movement of CO_2 from the bloodstream to the alveoli, where it is removed through exhalation

b. Gas exchange depends on tidal volume, the amount of air normally inhaled or exhaled

c. Not all of the tidal volume reaches the alveoli, where it can participate in gas exchange

d. Dead space refers to the portion of tidal volume remaining in those areas that conduct air but that are not involved in gas exchange; normally, this amount constitutes one-third of the tidal volume, but it may increase when physiologic dead space (areas that normally contribute to ventilation) and excessive tubing on mechanical ventilators are included

e. Gas exchange takes place on the surface of the alveoli

f. Alveolar type II cells secrete surfactant, a lipoprotein that decreases surface tension of the cell membrane and prevents alveolar collapse

g. Gas distribution to all lung areas is not uniform

h. The relationship of gas to blood flow is expressed as the ventilation/perfusion (V/Q) ratio and is normally 0.8 (4 liters/minute ventilation to 5 liters/minute perfusion)

i. When perfusion exists without ventilation, shunting occurs; the blood bypasses the alveoli and does not participate in gas exchange. Normally, this amounts to about 2% of inspired air but may be as high as 50% in disease states, such as adult respiratory distress syndrome

j. Insufficient O_2 exchange results in hypoxemia, and insufficient CO_2 exchange results in hypercarbia

k. The adequacy of gas exchange is determined by ABG analysis and mixed venous blood analysis

2. Regulation

a. Breathing is regulated by neurons in the medulla, by acid-base status, and by the state of wakefulness

b. Central chemoreceptors are sensitive to changes in the CO_2 level, which is the primary stimulus for breathing

c. Peripheral chemoreceptors are sensitive to changes in the O_2 level and in pH and provide a secondary stimulus for breathing

    d. Perfusion is regulated by cardiac output and obstruction to blood flow

    e. Gas exchange results from diffusion based on pressure gradients across the cell membrane

3. Application to critical care and emergency nursing

    a. Patients admitted to critical care or emergency areas commonly suffer from conditions that interfere with gas exchange

    b. Ineffective gas exchange leads to hypoxia, as evidenced by lactic acidosis, altered tissue perfusion, and organ dysfunction

    c. Knowledge of normal and abnormal laboratory and assessment findings is essential for managing a patient with inefficient gas exchange

    d. Patient care management is aimed at maintaining or improving gas exchange

Points to Remember

A steady balance (1:20) between acids and bases must be maintained for optimum cellular functioning.

Arterial blood pH is an indirect measurement of the hydrogen ion concentration.

Fluid movement is determined by cell membrane permeability, fluid osmolality, crystalloid and colloid osmotic pressure, and capillary hydrostatic pressure.

Adequate tissue perfusion is essential to adequate cellular functioning.

Changes in the CO_2 level are the primary stimulus for breathing.

O_2 is transported in the blood primarily by binding with hemoglobin.

Glossary

Capillary hydrostatic pressure—pressure of fluid against the blood vessel walls

Diffusion—passive movement of particles or solutes from an area of higher concentration to one of lower concentration

Electrolytes—active chemical particles, positively or negatively charged, that form varying combinations in body fluids; concentrations of electrolytes are commonly expressed in milliequivalents (mEq)

Osmosis—process of water movement across a semipermeable membrane in response to osmotic pressure; water moves from an area of lower solute concentration to one of higher concentration.

Surfactant—lipoprotein that decreases surface tension of the cell membrane and prevents alveolar collapse

Psychosocial Aspects of Critical Care and Emergency Nursing

Learning Objectives

After studying this section, the reader should be able to:

● Recognize general principles related to the psychosocial implications of critical and emergency illness.

● Name major problems that confront the patient and family during critical or emergency illness or hospitalization.

● Discuss common physical and behavioral assessment findings for the patient with impaired psychosocial integrity.

● Describe patient care management for the patient and family in crisis because of illness or hospitalization.

III. Psychosocial Aspects of Critical Care and Emergency Nursing

A. **Basic concepts**
1. In the cycle of health and illness, most patients go through three stages:
   a. A transition from health to illness when the patient and family experience denial, disbelief, or shock
   b. A developing awareness and acceptance that the patient needs help from others
   c. A reorganizational period when the patient's interest in life is renewed and he makes plans for the future
2. Critical or emergency illness alters a patient's sense of well-being, independence, and self-esteem as he faces the task of coping with the illness
3. The patient and family try to adapt to critical or emergency illness by using coping skills that differ in appropriateness and helpfulness
4. Most patients use previously employed coping patterns, either consciously or unconsciously, to deal with the environment and their situation
5. Factors that affect the patient's basic coping mechanisms result from exposure to stressors
   a. Biologic stressors include injury or illness, its severity, and the patient's perception of its significance
   b. Psychosocial stressors include interpersonal conflicts with family, legal or financial considerations, and growth and developmental conflicts
   c. Environmental stressors in the emergency department (ED) or intensive care unit (ICU) include unfamiliarity with the surroundings, sensory overload, sensory deprivation, and isolation
6. Patients in the ED or ICU experience psychosocial problems from fear, depression, powerlessness, sleep deprivation, or anxiety
7. Admission to an ED, and particularly to an ICU, causes a severe disruption in the patient's and family's routine; different surroundings, rules, smells, and people cause stress on the patient's territorial needs
8. The territorial needs of privacy, autonomy, self-identity, and security must be met; to meet these needs in a hospital, the patient establishes a temporary territory
9. When territoriality is overlooked by the nurse, the patient's feeling of lack of control may lead to anxiety
10. Signs of anxiety in the patient or family depend on the degree of anxiety experienced. Mild anxiety can heighten the use of coping skills; severe anxiety can incapacitate the patient
11. Patients and families face major problems during illness, which may occur simultaneously with or recur periodically during the illness. These include:
    a. Dealing with the symptoms, discomfort, and incapacitation of the illness or injury
    b. Managing the stress associated with treatments and hospitalization
    c. Developing and maintaining relationships with members of the medical team
    d. Maintaining a positive self-image and a sense of competence
    e. Dealing with the disturbing feelings evoked by illness or treatment

       f. Maintaining relationships with family and significant others despite role alterations

       g. Preparing for an uncertain future

  12. The universal need of families in crisis is hope

  13. Effective communication among the patient, family, and nurse is essential and can help:

       a. Reduce anxiety

       b. Identify health needs

       c. Clarify misconceptions

       d. Develop a supportive relationship

  14. Potential nursing diagnoses for a patient in crisis because of illness or hospitalization include:

       a. Anxiety

       b. Ineffective individual coping

       c. Disturbance in self-concept

       d. Spiritual distress

       e. Social isolation

       f. Sensory-perceptual alteration

       g. Ineffective family coping

       h. Altered family processes

B. Assessing the need for psychosocial intervention

   1. Physical assessment findings

       a. Increased muscle tension

       b. Increased perspiration, clammy skin

       c. Fatigue

       d. Restlessness

       e. Increased heart rate

       f. Increased rate or depth of respiration

       g. Diarrhea

       h. Urinary urgency

       i. Decreased appetite

       j. Dilated pupils

       k. Changes in body temperature or blood pressure

   2. Behavioral assessment findings

       a. Increased number of questions

       b. Increased verbalization of anxiety

       c. Increased focus on equipment or procedures

       d. Increased acting out

       e. Decreased focus on feelings

       f. Decreased ability to follow directions

C. Patient care management goal: to help the patient and family resolve the immediate problem, regain equilibrium, and resolve the overall crisis
1. Orient the patient and family to the environment to alleviate anxiety
2. Explain nursing actions and treatment
3. Give the patient personal and environmental control alternatives to alleviate feelings of powerlessness
4. Include family or support persons in explanations and care
5. Maintain appropriate wake and sleep cycles to encourage normal sleep patterns
6. Minimize conversation and equipment noise to prevent sensory overload
7. Provide information the patient needs to be effective in a given situation
8. Provide opportunities for private interactions between the patient and family
9. Help the patient and family to:
   a. Assess previous and present coping behaviors
   b. Identify strengths and positive coping behaviors
   c. Identify and minimize stressors
   d. Interact effectively with others
   e. Perform self-care activities
   f. Express appropriate concern for medical condition
   g. Actively participate in decisions regarding care, treatment, and the future

Points to Remember

Critical care and emergency nurses need to recognize anxiety and encourage the patient and family to express concerns and fears.

Most people use previously employed coping mechanisms to deal with a changed environment and an unfamiliar situation.

Denial, anger, withdrawal, and demanding behavior may reflect coping patterns used during critical and emergency illnesses.

Critical or emergency illness is a potential life crisis for the patient and family.

Glossary

Anxiety—vague, uneasy feeling caused by a nonspecific threat, real or imagined; the intensity of the feeling may range from mild to severe panic

Fear—feeling caused by a specific threat, real or imagined; the patient can identify the object of his fear; the intensity of the feeling may range from mild to severe panic

Powerlessness—perceived lack of control over a situation that an individual feels his actions cannot alter

Territoriality—desire or need to possess and occupy a space and, if necessary, to defend it against intrusion from others

Nutritional Support

Learning Objectives

After studying this section, the reader should be able to:

• Describe the general principles related to nutritional support.

• Identify physiologic changes caused by inadequate nutrition.

• Discuss the common physical assessment and diagnostic test findings related to inadequate nutrition.

• Describe care management for the patient receiving nutritional support.

IV. Nutritional Support

A. Basic concepts

1. Adequate nutrition exists when carbohydrates, proteins, fats, water, vitamins, and minerals are consumed in sufficient amounts to meet the body's metabolic requirements
2. The amount of nutrients needed to meet metabolic requirements is based on changes related to:
   a. Basal metabolic needs
   b. Activity
   c. Growth
   d. Health status
   e. Stress
3. Without a supply of dextrose, serum insulin levels drop, causing body fat to be used as energy; free fatty acids are mobilized from adipose tissue and are broken down in the liver to ketone bodies, causing ketosis
4. Inadequate nutrition causes the progressive loss of lean body mass and fat stores as the body's demands exceed its intake; this can lead to:
   a. Impaired wound healing
   b. Decreased resistance to infection
   c. Muscle wasting
   d. Inefficient cell-mediated immunity
   e. Decubitus ulcer formation
   f. Anemia
   g. Death
5. Risk factors for inadequate nutrition include:
   a. Age (infants, children, older adults)
   b. Recent illness or injury
   c. History of alcohol or drug abuse
   d. Severe trauma
   e. Serious infection
   f. Prolonged fever
   g. Massive burns
   h. Prolonged nausea, vomiting, diarrhea, wound drainage, or dialysis
6. Body weight is one of the most reliable indicators of nutritional status
7. Interpretation of weight trends in patients with unstable volume status may be difficult but must include:
   a. Intracellular fluid shifts
   b. Extracellular fluid shifts
   c. Diuresis
   d. Weight of dressing or equipment
8. Critically ill patients are at high risk for developing malnutrition because of conditions that limit intake or nutrient absorption or that increase nutritional demands
9. Many critically ill patients cannot meet nutritional requirements orally

10. Potential nursing diagnoses for the patient who needs nutritional support include:
    a. Altered nutrition: less than body requirements
    b. Potential for infection
    c. Impaired skin integrity

B. Types of nutritional support

1. Nutrients must be given in a form that is nutritionally acceptable, tolerated, and utilized; alternate methods of feeding include:
   a. Tube or enteral feedings
   b. Peripheral I.V. infusion
   c. Peripheral parenteral nutrition (PPN), which delivers nutrition through peripheral veins
   d. Total parenteral nutrition (TPN), which delivers nutrition through a central vein; formerly called hyperalimentation
   e. Parenteral lipid emulsions
2. The choice of nutritional support formula is based on its osmolality (the concentration of carbohydrates, amino acids, and electrolytes determines the osmolality of nutritional formulas)
   a. Isotonic solutions have about the same osmolality as blood (300 mOsm)
   b. Hypertonic or hyperosmolar solutions have a greater osmolality than blood. Enteral feedings administered too rapidly or before the patient has adjusted to the high concentration of particles can cause water to rush into the intestine and dilute the particles in concentration; this can lead to nausea, cramping, and diarrhea (dumping syndrome). Parenteral administration can cause fluid to move to the vascular compartment
3. The nutritional support formula chosen and the route of administration depend on:
   a. Nutritional needs
   b. Fluid tolerance
   c. Absorptive abilities of the GI tract
4. Enteral nutritional support given by the nasogastric, gastric, or jejunostomy route usually involves commercially prepared formulas:
   a. Iso-osmolar: providing about 1 calorie/ml; has the same osmolality as plasma
   b. Hyperosmolar: providing about 1 to 2 calories/ml; high osmolality makes this type of formula less tolerated
   c. Elemental: providing specific nutrient components with high osmolality; best tolerated if administered into the small bowel
   d. Special formulas: restricting protein, sodium, or potassium; given to patients with renal or liver disease
5. Parenteral nutritional support is given through a peripheral or central I.V. line.
   a. Peripheral I.V. solutions consist of water with glucose, electrolytes, or both; they are used short-term because they have little nutritional or caloric value

    b. PPN solutions are administered through a peripheral I.V. line and consist of an isotonic or hypotonic infusion of dextrose (5% to 10%), amino acids (3% to 8.5%), vitamins, electrolytes, and trace elements; they provide temporary nutritional support to promote nitrogen balance and weight gain when the enteral route is inadequate or contraindicated or during transition from TPN to enteral intake

    c. TPN solutions are administered through a central I.V. line and consist of a hypertonic complete nutrition solution of dextrose (25% to 70%), amino acids (3.5% to 10%), vitamins, electrolytes, and trace elements; their composition depends on the patient's nutritional needs and clinical condition. They provide complete nutritional support when the enteral route is inadequate or contraindicated

    d. Parenteral lipid emulsions consist of essential fatty acids (10% or 20%); isotonic fat emulsion can contribute up to 60% of the total daily calorie intake to correct or prevent essential fatty acid deficiency. These emulsions are usually recommended in combination with TPN or PPN but can be used by themselves to replace carbohydrate calories in patients with glucose intolerance or when carbon dioxide (CO_2) production must be avoided

C. Assessing the need for nutritional support

  1. Physical assessment findings

    a. Weight: recent unplanned weight loss equaling 10% or more of normal weight

    b. Anthropometric measurement: triceps skinfold and mid-upper-arm muscle circumference measurements less than standard

    c. Tissue wasting

    d. Hair loss

    e. Delayed wound healing

    f. Petechiae

    g. Ecchymoses

  2. Diagnostic test findings

    a. Nitrogen balance: negative

    b. Serum albumin levels: less than 4 g/dl

    c. Serum transferrin levels: less than 250 mcg/dl

    d. Hemoglobin: less than 12 g/dl (female); less than 14 g/dl (male)

    e. Hematocrit: less than 37% (female); less than 45% (male)

    f. Total protein levels: less than 6 g/dl

    g. Urine urea nitrogen levels: increased nitrogen (in early inadequate nutritional states); decreased nitrogen (in late inadequate nutritional states)

D. **Patient care management goal (enteral route): to maintain lean body mass and to provide adequate nutrients and energy to sustain physiologic processes**
1. Perform a nutritional assessment
   a. Monitor serum diagnostic tests for abnormalities
   b. Obtain triceps skinfold and mid-upper-arm muscle measurements and compare to standards; measurements are typically difficult to obtain in critically ill patients
   c. Perform a 24-hour dietary recall and calorie counts
2. Assess the placement and function of the feeding tube
   a. Check the position of the large-bore tube by injecting air while listening over the stomach with a stethoscope or by aspirating gastric contents
   b. Do not initiate tube feeding through a small-bore tube until the tube's position has been documented by X-ray
3. Assess for intolerance to formula, as evidenced by stool frequency and consistency, nausea or vomiting, gastric residual, and abdominal distention
4. Raise the head of the bed 30 degrees, if possible, to enhance gravity flow; maintain this position for 1 hour after feeding
5. Check the gastric residual by aspirating stomach content
   a. If the residual is greater than 100 ml, return the aspirate and notify the doctor, or follow institutional policy on continuation of feeding
   b. If the residual is less than 100 ml, return the aspirate and continue feeding
6. Assess fluid and hydration status
   a. Record input and output (I/O), assessing 24-hour trends
   b. Weigh the patient daily at the same time with the same scale
7. Monitor for diarrhea, which may be caused by problems with the formula administration
   a. If the feeding rate is too fast, start feeding at 50 ml/hour and increase by 25 ml/hr every 8 to 12 hours, depending on the patient's tolerance or the doctor's order
   b. If the formula volume is too great, decrease it to a level tolerated by the patient, gradually increasing it as tolerated; feed smaller volumes at more frequent intervals. Use a continuous-drip method of administration
   c. If the formula is too cold, administer it at room temperature
   d. Give initial feeding of hypertonic formula at one-third to one-half the rate for a minimum of 8 hours, gradually increasing the concentration; do not increase rate and strength at the same time
   e. If the patient has a low serum albumin level (decreased oncotic pressure causes increased water in the bowel, leading to diarrhea), dilute the formula and increase the concentration gradually
8. Institute measures to prevent bacterial contamination of the formula and equipment
   a. Wash hands before handling equipment
   b. Administer the formula promptly after opening; do not add newly opened formula to formula in the bag

      c. Replace the feeding bag and tubing according to institutional policy

      d. Cover and date the unused formula and store it in the refrigerator; use it within 24 hours or as recommended by manufacturer

      e. Do not allow continuous-drip feedings to hang longer than 8 hours

      f. Rinse equipment before and after feeding

  9. Assess the patient for regurgitation of stomach contents, leading to potential aspiration pneumonia

      a. Elevate the head of the bed 30 degrees for at least 1 hour after feeding to ensure proper feeding position

      b. If the patient experiences slowed gastric emptying time (gastric residual greater than 100 ml), check the gastric residual before each intermittent feeding and every 4 hours with the continuous-delivery method

      c. If the gastroesophageal sphincter becomes incompetent from the large-bore feeding tube, change to a feeding tube with a smaller diameter

      d. Check the tube position every shift to prevent improper placement

10. Assess for complaints of nausea

      a. Explain the procedure to the patient to allay his anxiety, providing him time for questions and emotional support

      b. Check the tube for proper placement

      c. Decrease the rate of feeding or use the continuous-drip method if the feeding rate is too rapid

      d. If the volume is too great or gastric emptying is delayed, reduce the rate and then increase it gradually; check the gastric residual and, if greater than 100 ml, replace aspirated residual and follow institutional policy. Encourage ambulation if distention is a problem

      e. Notify the doctor of any intolerance to a specific formula so that he can consider changing to another formula

11. Assess for possible fluid volume imbalances

      a. Assess trends in I/O, checking for alternate reasons for fluid gain or loss

      b. Check for excess water entering the feeding tube from rinsing the tube or administering medication

      c. Monitor for excessive protein intake, which can increase urine output; evaluate the patient's protein requirements, increasing fluid intake if possible

12. Maintain feeding tube patency

      a. Flush the tube before and after each feeding with 30 to 50 ml of water

      b. Completely dissolve medications before administration, or use liquid medications and flush with water after administration

      c. Note that a small-bore feeding tube may not deliver high-viscosity formulas efficiently; instead, infuse these formulas by pump or notify the doctor so he can consider low-viscosity formulas

E. Patient care management goal (parenteral route): to maintain lean body mass and to provide adequate nutrients and energy to sustain physiologic processes

  1. Perform a nutritional assessment

      a. Obtain serum diagnostic tests for abnormalities

    b. Assess triceps skinfold and mid-upper-arm muscle measurements and compare with standards

    c. Perform a 24-hour dietary recall and calorie counts

    d. Obtain the patient's weight and compare it to baseline

2. Maintain aseptic technique, using thorough hand washing before touching to prevent infection

3. Record I/O, assessing 24-hour trends to prevent fluid imbalances

4. Control infusion rate with an I.V. pump to prevent fluid overload

5. Observe for complications of TPN, including sepsis, line occlusion, glucose intolerance, and fungal infection

6. Minimize the risk of infection to the patient with TPN

    a. Do not use the TPN line to give blood, administer medications, or measure central venous pressure

    b. Allow the TPN solution to hang for no more than 24 hours; use a filter to prevent infusion of gross particles

    c. Keep the TPN solution refrigerated until administration, and check the label on fluids for correct name and concentrations

    d. Change the catheter and dressing according to institutional policy

7. Monitor fluid and electrolyte levels to prevent possible imbalances

    a. Start the infusion rate slowly to allow the patient's body to adapt to the high glucose load and osmolality; gradually increase the rate as ordered until the desired rate is achieved

    b. If the infusion falls behind, do not attempt to compensate by adjusting it to a higher-than-desired rate; hyperosmolar diuresis may result from excessive glucose infusion

    c. Gradually wean the patient from TPN to prevent rebound hypoglycemia; use a dextrose 10% solution temporarily if replacement TPN solution is not readily available from the pharmacy

    d. Monitor serum electrolyte levels to prevent imbalances; obtain fingerstick blood glucose levels to detect hyperglycemia

    e. Remember that the end-product of carbohydrate metabolism is CO_2, which may cause increasing $PaCO_2$ levels in patients with respiratory compromise

8. Administer lipid emulsions, as ordered, to correct fatty acid deficiency

    a. Do not give I.V. lipids to patients with abnormal lipid metabolism, severe liver disease, or acute pancreatitis

    b. Check the manufacturer's directions for lipid emulsion storage; let refrigerated emulsion stand at room temperature for 30 minutes before hanging

    c. Do not shake fat emulsions to prevent separation

    d. Hang the fat emulsion with the TPN solution, according to institutional policy, connected beyond the filter and as close to the insertion site as possible

Points to Remember

Critically ill patients are at high risk for inadequate nutrition from conditions that increase nutritional demands or limit nutrient intake or absorption.

Body weight is one of the most reliable indicators of nutritional status.

Enteral feedings may be administered by the continuous-drip method or by intermittent bolus feedings.

Complications associated with TPN include sepsis, glucose intolerance, line occlusion, and fungal infection.

Glossary

Gastric residual—amount of stomach contents that remains and is aspirated by a feeding syringe; the amount indicates the effectiveness of gastric absorption

Ketosis—accumulation of ketone bodies in body tissues and fluids caused by the breakdown of fatty acids

Negative nitrogen balance—catabolic state in which more nitrogen is excreted than taken in

Osmolality—concentration of a solution based on the number of particles in the solution

Infection Control

Learning Objectives

After studying this section, the reader should be able to:

- Describe the general principles related to infection control.

- Identify the common causes of infection in the critically ill patient.

- Discuss the common physical assessment and diagnostic test findings used to determine the need for infection control.

- Describe care management for the patient with an infection.

V. Infection Control

A. Basic concepts

1. Although all patients must be protected from infection, patients with active infections are most in need of infection control measures
2. Critically ill patients are at grave risk for infection because their immune systems are commonly debilitated and severely compromised
3. The most common infection sites in the critically ill patient are the urinary tract, the respiratory tract, the wound site, and the blood
4. The most common cause of primary bacteremia (sepsis) is the insertion of intravascular devices
   a. Critically ill patients typically require the placement of central or peripheral vein access lines for hemodynamic monitoring
   b. Bacteremia acquired in the critical care unit usually originates from the insertion of intravascular catheters
5. Nearly 50% of the patients who acquire septicemia are likely to die as a result
   a. Septicemia can occur in patients of all ages
   b. Septicemia can occur in acutely and chronically ill patients
6. Certain disease processes, such as diabetes, severe trauma, renal failure, chronic lung disease, and leukemia, predispose the patient to an increased risk for infection
7. The patient admitted on an emergency basis may be unable to communicate previous exposure to or presence of infectious disease
8. Concern over life-threatening illness may take precedence over suspected infectious disease
9. The patient being treated for one infection may develop a secondary infection from exposure in the hospital or from antibiotic therapy
10. Potential nursing diagnoses for a patient with an infection include:
    a. Altered tissue perfusion
    b. Social isolation
    c. Knowledge deficit

B. Assessing the need for infection control

1. Physical assessment findings
   a. Symptoms may be masked or absent if the patient is immunosuppressed or receiving antibiotics
   b. Local symptoms depend on the infection site and may include inflammation, redness, and purulent drainage
   c. Systemic symptoms may include fever, chills, and tachycardia
2. Diagnostic test findings
   a. White blood cell (WBC) count: elevated unless the causative organism is viral or mycoplasmic

    b. WBC differential: increased number of neutrophils as evidence that the body is fighting infection

    c. Culture and sensitivity studies: identify the organism and reveal the appropriate antibiotic to use for treatment

C. Patient care management goal: to prevent or treat infection

1. Obtain diagnostic studies to identify the cause or source of the infection
   a. Diagnostic studies are valid only if the specimen is properly collected, transported, and processed
   b. Collection protocols may vary among institutions
   c. To prevent contamination, strict sterile technique is required when collecting any specimen to be studied for culture
2. Administer drugs, as ordered
   a. Antibiotics appropriate to the organism are given at specified times, according to pharmacologic recommendations for the presence or absence of food in the gut, to maintain adequate blood levels
   b. Evaluation of the patient's renal and liver function is essential to determine the correct dosage
   c. Resistant organisms may require frequent adjustments in choice and dosage of drugs
   d. Appropriate drugs treat the underlying pathophysiologic process contributing to the infection; these include insulin for diabetes and bronchodilators for chronic lung disease
3. Wear gloves any time skin or mucous membrane is likely to come in contact with blood or other body fluids
   a. Procedures likely to cause contamination from excreta include suctioning, dressing changes, urine measurement, toileting, and obtaining blood specimens
   b. Precautions protect the patient and the nurse
4. Wash hands, using vigorous friction, under running water with standard soap; this is the primary means of preventing infection
   a. Antiseptic soaps should be used in high-risk clinical areas
   b. Hands should be washed between contact with different patients, between different procedures on the same patient, and before and after gloves are worn (skin flora multiply rapidly in gloves)
5. Adhere strictly to protocols for catheter insertion and care to markedly reduce catheter-related infections
   a. Use of any catheter (urinary or vascular) must be essential for care and not a convenience for the medical or nursing staff
   b. Any catheter must be inserted under strict sterile conditions
   c. Site care must be performed according to guidelines from the Centers for Disease Control (CDC) and institutional policy
   d. All connection sites are potential sources of contamination; the catheter system should be manipulated only after strict hand washing or donning gloves

6. Decrease risks of infection by adhering to established guidelines
   a. Sharing of equipment between patients should be avoided
   b. Equipment needing careful decontamination includes that which cannot be autoclaved, such as transducers, monitor parts, and oxygen and ventilator equipment
   c. Spills, especially blood and other excreta, should be removed immediately
   d. Personnel with active infections, especially upper respiratory infections and herpetic lesions, should be restricted from patient contact
7. Care for infection sites properly
   a. Dressings should be changed as frequently as necessary to keep the site clean and dry
   b. Cross-contamination of sites is prevented by covering each area with a separate dressing
   c. Wound care varies according to site, infective organism, and institutional policy
8. Prevent transmission of infection by following the CDC's isolation guidelines
9. Separate patients with a diagnosed infection, if possible, from other patients in the critical care unit to prevent cross-contamination
10. Provide patient teaching to assist in:
    a. Identifying risk factors and causative agents contributing to the infection
    b. Describing the importance of adhering to specific drug regimens for treatment
    c. Recognizing the importance of informing others of infection if it will have a major health impact, such as with hepatitis, herpes, or acquired immunodeficiency syndrome

Points to Remember

Intravascular catheter-related sepsis is the primary cause of septicemia in the critically ill patient.

Nearly 50% of patients who become septic are likely to die as a result.

Proper hand washing is the primary means to prevent infection transmission.

Gloves are indicated to prevent skin and mucous membrane exposure to blood and body fluids.

Patients should be strongly encouraged to inform others of a history of infection if it will have a major impact on health or life-style practices.

Glossary

Catheter-related sepsis—systemic infection that can occur from the insertion and placement of an indwelling catheter

Cross-contamination—spread of infective organisms from one site or person to another

Resistant organism—organism that is insensitive to a prescribed antibiotic

Septicemia—systemic disease process caused by microorganisms and their toxic products in the blood

Emergency Life Support: Resuscitation

Learning Objectives

After studying this section, the reader should be able to:

● Describe the general principles related to the patient requiring resuscitation.

● Identify the common causes of cardiopulmonary arrest.

● Discuss the common physical assessment and diagnostic test findings used to determine the need for resuscitation.

● Describe care management for the patient requiring resuscitation.

VI. Emergency Life Support: Resuscitation

A. Basic concepts

1. Cardiopulmonary resuscitation (CPR) is indicated for cardiac arrest
   a. Cardiac arrest occurs when the heart stops beating (asystole) or when contractions are inadequate to maintain cardiac output, as in ventricular tachycardia or fibrillation
   b. Cardiac arrest may be precipitated by myocardial infarction (most common), heart failure, shock, severe electrolyte imbalance, acid-base imbalance, drowning, electrocution, drug overdose, or respiratory arrest
   c. Cardiac arrest is always accompanied immediately by respiratory arrest
   d. Respiratory arrest may be precipitated by airway obstruction, acute exacerbation of chronic airway disease, status asthmaticus, or drug overdose
   e. Respiratory arrest, if untreated, will precipitate cardiac arrest
2. Life support, or CPR, follows an A-B-C sequence
   a. A—open the *airway* by lifting the jaw and tilting the head back (unless a neck injury is present)
   b. B—restore *breathing* by artificial ventilation (mouth-to-mouth resuscitation or a ventilatory assist device)
   c. C—restore *circulation* by delivering closed chest compressions
3. The American Heart Association (AHA) designates two types of emergency life support
   a. Basic cardiac life support (BCLS) is emergency first aid focused on identifying respiratory or cardiac arrest and providing CPR until the victim responds or the next type of life support is initiated
   b. Advanced cardiac life support (ACLS) includes BCLS plus the use of adjunctive therapies to support ventilation, such as establishment of I.V. lifelines, drug administration, cardiac monitoring, defibrillation, control of dysrhythmias, and postresuscitation care
4. Optimal responses are achieved if BCLS is initiated within 4 minutes of the cardiac arrest followed by ACLS within 8 minutes of the arrest
5. Specific procedures for BCLS and ACLS are defined by the AHA's Standards and Guidelines for Cardiopulmonary Resuscitation and Emergency Cardiac Care
6. All health professionals should be competent in BCLS skills
7. All doctors and nurses practicing in critical care and emergency areas must be competent in ACLS skills
8. Potential nursing diagnoses for a patient requiring resuscitation include:
   a. Altered cardiac output
   b. Altered tissue perfusion
   c. Ineffective breathing pattern

B. Assessing the need for life support

1. Physical assessment findings
   a. Unresponsiveness
   b. Gasping or absent respiration

COMMON LIFE-SUPPORT DRUGS

DRUG	INDICATIONS	PRECAUTIONS
atropine sulfate	Bradycardia, asystole	• Lower dose (less than 0.5 mg) may cause bradycardia. • Higher dose (more than 2 mg) may cause full vagal blockage. • Contraindicated for glaucoma patients (use isoproterenol instead).
bretylium tosylate (Bretylate, Bretylol)	Life-threatening ventricular fibrillation and ventricular tachycardia	• Generally not used to treat premature ventricular contractions unless other drugs fail. • May increase digitalis toxicity. • May lower blood pressure.
dobutamine hydrochloride (Dobutrex)	Acute congestive heart failure, cardiopulmonary bypass surgery	• Don't use with beta blockers, such as propranolol. • Patients with atrial fibrillation should receive digoxin first, or they can develop rapid ventricular response. • Drug is incompatible with alkaline solutions. • Infiltration may produce severe tissue damage.
dopamine hydrochloride (Intropin)	Shock, decreased renal function	• Don't use for treating uncorrected tachydysrhythmias or ventricular fibrillation. • May precipitate dysrhythmias. • Drug is incompatible with alkaline solutions. • Infiltration may produce severe tissue damage. • Solution deteriorates after 24 hours.
epinephrine hydrochloride (Adrenalin)	Bronchospasm, anaphylaxis, severe allergic reactions, cardiac arrest, dysrhythmias	• Increases intraocular pressure. • May exacerbate congestive heart failure, dysrhythmias, angina pectoris, hyperthyroidism, and emphysema. • May cause headache, tremors, or palpitations.
isoproterenol hydrochloride (Isuprel)	Bronchospasm, cardiac dysrhythmias, cardiac arrest	• Don't administer with epinephrine. • Don't mix with barbiturates, sodium bicarbonate, any calcium preparation, or aminophylline.
lidocaine hydrochloride (Xylocaine)	Ventricular dysrhythmias	• Don't mix with sodium bicarbonate. • Don't use if patient has high-grade sinoatrial or atrioventricular (AV) block. • Discontinue if PR interval or QRS complex widens or if dysrhythmias worsen. • May lead to CNS toxicity.

COMMON LIFE-SUPPORT DRUGS continued

DRUG	INDICATIONS	PRECAUTIONS
procainamide hydrochloride (Pronestyl)	Dysrhythmias, malignant hyperthermia	• Can cause precipitous hypotension; don't use for treating second- or third-degree heart block unless a pacemaker has been inserted. • Can cause AV block.
sodium bicarbonate	Metabolic acidosis, cardiac arrest	• Don't mix with epinephrine; causes epinephrine degradation. • Don't mix with calcium salts; forms insoluble precipitates.
verapamil hydrochloride (Calan, Isoptin)	Supraventricular tachydysrhythmias, angina, hypertension	• Contraindicated in patients with hypotension, cardiogenic shock, severe congestive heart failure, or second- or third-degree AV block. • High doses or administering too rapidly can cause a significant drop in blood pressure.

    c. Lack of palpable carotid pulse
    d. Lack of audible or palpable blood pressure
    e. Dysrhythmia, which may include ventricular tachycardia or fibrillation, asystole, or electromechanical disassociation
  2. Diagnostic test findings
    a. Arterial blood gas (ABG) analysis: respiratory acidosis and hypoxemia
    b. ECG: ventricular tachycardia or fibrillation, asystole
    c. Serum potassium levels: below or above normal; may precipitate dysrhythmias
    d. Serum calcium levels: low in patients on calcium channel blockers

C. Patient care management goal: to restore effective breathing and cardiac output
  1. Initiate BCLS and ACLS according to AHA guidelines
    a. Cardiac monitoring to identify dysrhythmias
    b. Defibrillation by authorized personnel
    c. Intubation and oxygen administration to support ventilation
    d. I.V. lifeline access—peripheral or central site—for administration of drugs and fluids
    e. Drug therapy to treat cardiac dysrhythmias, decreased cardiac output, and acid-base imbalances

2. Follow institutional policies that determine nursing responsibilities in ACLS protocols
3. Document the therapy sequence and responses to therapy according to institutional policy
4. Support the family and help them prepare to see the patient by describing:
   a. Changes in his appearance
   b. Presence and purpose of endotracheal, nasogastric, or I.V. tubes
5. Provide patient teaching to assist him in:
   a. Identifying the risk factors and causative agents that may have contributed to his cardiopulmonary arrest
   b. Discussing the fear and anxiety he may have felt because of a near-death experience
   c. Recognizing the importance of having family members trained in BCLS

Points to Remember

Life support, or CPR, follows an A-B-C sequence: A—airway; B—breathing; C—circulation

Optimal responses from resuscitation are achieved if BCLS is initiated within 4 minutes—followed by ACLS within 8 minutes—of the cardiac arrest.

The most common cause of sudden cardiac arrest is myocardial infarction.

Family members of high-risk patients should learn to initiate BCLS.

Glossary

ACLS—emergency first aid that includes BCLS plus the use of drugs and adjunctive therapies, such as ventilation and defibrillation, to restore cardiac function

BCLS—emergency first aid focusing on identifying respiratory or cardiac arrest and providing CPR

CPR—cardiopulmonary resuscitation, which includes both mouth-to-mouth breathing and closed cardiac compressions

Defibrillation—electrical therapy used to terminate chaotic cardiac activity and reestablish a normal rhythm

Mechanical Ventilation

Learning Objectives

After studying this section, the reader should be able to:

- Describe the general principles of mechanical ventilation.

- Identify the different types of mechanical ventilators.

- Describe the mode of action for the common types of ventilators.

- Describe diagnostic test findings that support mechanical ventilation

- Discuss the measures used to wean a patient from mechanical ventilation.

- Describe care management for the patient requiring mechanical ventilation.

VII. Mechanical Ventilation

A. Basic concepts

1. Mechanical ventilation is the artificial support of or assistance to breathing when the patient cannot provide an adequate gas exchange to supply his body tissues with oxygen
   a. Takes over the physical work of moving air in and out of the lungs
   b. Does not replace or alter physiologic lung function
2. The ventilator is connected to an artificial airway
   a. An oral or nasal endotracheal (ET) tube is used for short-term ventilation (cuffed for adults and uncuffed for children)
   b. A tracheostomy tube is used for long-term ventilation
3. Mechanical ventilation is used to:
   a. Provide mechanical power for the pulmonary system to maintain physiologic ventilation when the patient cannot breathe because of a neurologic or neuromuscular condition or a pharmacologically induced paralysis
   b. Improve the efficiency of ventilation or oxygenation by manipulating the ventilatory pattern and airway pressures
   c. Provide hyperventilation in the patient with head injuries
4. Complications of mechanical ventilation include:
   a. Pneumothorax—can occur because of alveolar rupture from the high positive pressure required to deliver a preset volume
   b. Barotrauma—can occur because of increased intrathoracic pressure that damages major vessels or organs in the thorax
   c. Alteration in hemodynamic pressures—can occur because of increased intrathoracic pressure that may impede venous return and lead to decreased cardiac output and increased pulmonary artery wedge pressure
   d. Increased intracranial pressure—can occur because of decreased venous return and blood pooling in the cerebral vessels
   e. Water imbalance—can occur because of humidified air use, reduced lymphatic flow, or syndrome of inappropriate antidiuretic hormone
5. Equipment and techniques for weaning the patient from mechanical ventilation include:
   a. IMV—the ventilatory rate is gradually decreased as the patient is able to resume the work of breathing; usually best for the patient on long-term ventilatory support
   b. T-piece adaptor placed on an ET tube with supplemental oxygen—the patient is taken off the ventilator and expected to breathe spontaneously for increasing periods before being returned to the ventilator to permit him to rest; usually used for patients ventilated to produce pharmacologic paralysis for a short procedure or for a short time postoperatively until anesthetic effects have worn off

6. Potential nursing diagnoses for a patient requiring mechanical ventilation include:
   a. Ineffective airway clearance
   b. Anxiety
   c. Ineffective breathing pattern
   d. Impaired gas exchange
   e. Potential for infection
   f. Impaired verbal communication
   g. Activity intolerance

B. Types and modes of ventilation
1. Ventilator type and mode are selected by the doctor based on the patient's specific needs and diagnosis
2. Types of ventilators include:
   a. Negative pressure—exerts negative pressure on the external chest (iron lung or cuirass); does not require intubation; is rarely used today
   b. Positive pressure, pressure-cycled—exerts positive pressure on the airway; a predetermined pressure terminates inspiration and may prohibit delivery of tidal volume if airway resistance is high
   c. Positive pressure, time-cycled—exerts positive pressure on the airway; delivers a volume of gas over a predetermined time
   d. Positive pressure, volume-cycled—exerts positive pressure on the airway; delivers a predetermined volume of gas and allows limits to be set for pressure and time; the most widely used ventilator
   e. Positive pressure, jet ventilation—exerts positive pressure on the airway; delivers small volumes of gas at very high rates
3. Modes of ventilation include:
   a. *Controlled mandatory ventilation (CMV)*—delivers a preset tidal volume at a preset rate, ignoring the patient's own ventilatory effort; the least frequently used mode of ventilation
   b. *Assist controlled ventilation (ACV)*—delivers a preset tidal volume for every breath initiated by the machine or through the patient's effort; allows hyperventilation
   c. *Intermittent mandatory ventilation (IMV)*—delivers a preset tidal volume at a preset rate while allowing the patient to breathe at his own rate and tidal volume; can cause breath stacking because the ventilation is delivered at a preset frequency and may not occur in the same phase as the patient's own efforts
   d. *Synchronized intermittent mandatory ventilation (SIMV)*—delivers a preset, mandatory tidal volume synchronized to the patient's inspiratory effort; the most widely used and therapeutic mode of ventilation
4. Ventilatory adjuncts include:
   a. Positive end-expiratory pressure (PEEP)—positive pressure exerted by mechanical ventilation at the end of expiration; used to counteract small airway collapse and facilitate gas exchange to improve oxygenation

    b. Continuous positive airway pressure (CPAP)—positive pressure exerted continuously by mechanical ventilation; may be used for spontaneously breathing patients to prevent alveolar collapse

5. Ventilator controls include:
   a. Mode—selection of CMV, ACV, IMV, or SIMV
   b. FIO_2—the fraction of inspired oxygen; usually reported as a percentage, although technically a decimal (.40 = 40%)
   c. Tidal volume—the amount of air in a normal breath, measured on inspiration or expiration; the amount of tidal volume set on a ventilator is 10 to 15 ml/kg of body weight
   d. Rate—the number of ventilator breaths delivered each minute; the patient's spontaneous rate is added to the ventilator rate to obtain the actual respiratory rate per minute
   e. Peak inspiratory pressure—the amount of pressure exerted to deliver a preset volume; limits are set to prevent barotrauma; remaining volume will not be delivered when pressure limit is reached
   f. Alarms—the safety devices used to monitor alterations in rate, volume, and pressure; these vary from machine to machine

C. Assessing the need for mechanical ventilation

1. Physical assessment findings
   a. Dyspnea
   b. Tachypnea
   c. Adventitious or absent breath sounds
   d. Cyanosis
   e. Alteration in mental status
   f. Tachycardia or other dysrhythmia as a result of hypoxia
2. Diagnostic test findings
   a. Arterial blood gas (ABG) levels: $PaCO_2$ greater than 50; PaO_2 less than 50; pH less than 7.35
   b. Tidal volume: less than 5 ml/kg
   c. Negative inspiratory force: less than -20 cm H_2O
   d. Minute volume (tidal volume $\times$ rate): less than 10 liters/minute

D. Patient care management goal: to decrease the work of breathing to improve gas exchange and tissue perfusion

1. Verify and maintain the ventilator settings according to the doctor's order and institutional policy
   a. Mode
   b. FIO_2
   c. Tidal volume
   d. Rate
   e. Ventilatory adjuncts, such as PEEP and CPAP
   f. Alarms

2. Suction as necessary to remove secretions
   a. Hyperoxygenate and hyperventilate before suctioning to prevent hypoxia
   b. Observe the patient carefully for decreases in heart rate during suctioning
3. Assess and document the following parameters: continuous ECG rhythm; vital signs; mental status; heart, lung, and bowel sounds; urine output; and any symptoms that indicate changes in these parameters
4. Assess and document hemodynamic status and pressures if a pulmonary artery catheter is in place
5. Administer drug therapy, as ordered:
   a. Bronchodilators to dilate smooth muscle of large airways
   b. Paralyzing agents, such as pancuronium bromide, to further decrease the work of breathing and maximize the use of mechanical ventilation
   c. Sedatives (always given with paralyzing agents) to decrease anxiety
   d. Diuretics to reduce circulating fluid and volume overload
   e. Antibiotics appropriate for the causative organism if infection is present
6. Insert a nasogastric tube to relieve gastric distention and prevent aspiration
7. Administer parenteral nutrition to support the patient's metabolic needs and defend against infection
8. Monitor ABG levels for hypoxia and acid-base imbalance to determine adequacy of ventilation
9. Place the patient in low- or semi-Fowler's position to improve comfort and to facilitate respiration
10. Troubleshoot *high-pressure ventilator alarms,* which may indicate that:
    a. Patient requires suctioning
    b. Tubing is kinked
    c. Water or secretions are in tubing
    d. Patient is biting ET tube
    e. Patient has bronchospasm or cough
    f. Patient has decreased lung compliance requiring higher inspiratory pressures
11. Troubleshoot *low-pressure ventilator alarms,* which may indicate that:
    a. Tubing is disconnected from machine circuit or from patient
    b. ET tube cuff has a leak
12. Apply soft restraints, if necessary, to protect the patient from self-extubation; use them according to institutional policy
13. Offer frequent mouth care and comfort measures while the patient is intubated
14. Communicate by asking questions that require a simple "yes" or "no" response, by gesturing, and by using a word or letter board
15. Assess for readiness to wean
    a. Negative inspiratory force: greater than -20 cm H_2O
    b. Tidal volume: greater than 15 ml/kg

    c. FIO_2: less than 40%

    d. ABG levels: $PaCO_2$ of 45 mm Hg or less; PaO_2 of 60 mm Hg or greater; and a pH of 7.35 to 7.45

16. Provide emotional support to decrease the patient's fear and anxiety
17. Provide patient teaching to assist him in
    a. Cooperating with the medical or nursing interventions to support breathing
    b. Recognizing the importance of frequently assessing level of consciousness and specimens for laboratory analysis
    c. Responding appropriately to nursing and family coaching on breathing techniques
    d. Recognizing the severity of his disease and the possible need for long-term ventilatory support

Points to Remember

Mechanical ventilation takes over the physical work of breathing but does not alter physiologic lung function.

Positive-pressure, volume-cycled ventilators are the most commonly used ventilators for adults.

Synchronized intermittent mandatory ventilation (SIMV) provides the most therapeutic mode of mechanical ventilation.

Pneumothorax is a common complication of mechanical ventilation.

Hyperoxygenation and hyperventilation before suctioning decrease the risk of hypoxia

Glossary

FIO$_2$ (fraction of inspired oxygen)—ventilator setting that refers to the fraction of inspired oxygen; actually a decimal but usually recorded as a percentage

NIF (negative inspiratory force)—measurement to demonstrate the muscle power needed to provide a tidal volume of 5 ml/kg; must be greater than -20 cm H$_2$O for spontaneous breathing to meet bodily needs

PEEP (positive end-expiratory pressure)—pressure exerted by mechanical ventilation at the end of expiration that keeps alveoli and small airways open to promote gas exchange

Pneumothorax—condition characterized by free air in the thoracic cavity, usually in the pleura, that has escaped from an opening in lung tissue; can result in tension pneumothorax with positive pressure ventilation and lead to mediastinal shift, which imposes on the unaffected lung and vascular structures

Tidal volume—amount of air breathed in or out with each breath

Hemodynamic Monitoring

Learning Objectives

After studying this section, the reader should be able to:

• Identify the basic principles of hemodynamic monitoring.

• List the information obtained through hemodynamic monitoring.

• Discuss the primary uses for each type of hemodynamic monitoring.

• Discuss the implications of readings obtained for each type of hemodynamic monitoring.

• Describe patient care management for each type of hemodynamic monitoring.

VIII. Hemodynamic Monitoring

A. Basic concepts
1. Hemodynamic pressures exist within the heart and the arterial system
2. Each chamber of the heart and the arterial system has normal pressures that can be measured and, with the use of a transducer, transformed into distinct waveforms
3. Insertion of a catheter into an artery or the heart enables the doctor and nurse to compare a patient's waveforms to normal values and to the patient's baseline values
4. Hemodynamic monitoring can be used to:
   a. Monitor various cardiovascular pressures directly
   b. Guide nursing interventions for the assessment of fluid status and the titration of drugs
   c. Assess treatment effectiveness by evaluating trends in obtained values
   d. Monitor the patient's progress continuously by evaluating pressure waveforms and values
5. General patient care management includes the following:
   a. Hemodynamic monitoring requires an informed consent
   b. Assess the patient's level of understanding of the rationale for catheter insertion, and prepare a teaching plan
   c. Set up the equipment according to institutional policy to prepare for insertion; aseptic technique is essential for line insertion and maintenance
   d. Observe the patient for anxiety and signs and symptoms of complications
   e. Assess the results of therapeutic interventions, and make ordered changes to fluids, drug therapy, or treatment measures
   f. Record pressure data and vital signs according to the patient's condition and institutional policy
   g. Level, zero, and calibrate the equipment to ensure accurate data at least once a shift or when values are questionable; level the transducer to the phlebostatic axis
   h. Maintain a fluid-filled pressure system to ensure accurate transmission of the pressure signal
   i. Change pressure system fluids, tubing, and dressings according to institutional policy
   j. Assess the patient and waveforms frequently for changes from the baseline assessment to prevent complications; these changes are regarded as trends
   k. Notify the doctor when parameters are outside acceptable ranges

B. Arterial pressure monitoring
1. General information
   a. Arterial pressure may be measured indirectly with a blood pressure cuff and stethoscope or with an automatic blood pressure–measuring device

b. Direct intra-arterial measurement may be taken after inserting a cannula into an artery connected to a pressure-monitoring device (intra-arterial monitoring is discussed in this section)

c. The catheter is inserted through the radial, brachial, or femoral artery

d. The radial artery is the preferred insertion site because the artery is small and superficial, with good collateral circulation

e. The brachial artery is a less desirable insertion site because the artery is deeper and more difficult to cannulate

f. The femoral artery is the least desirable insertion site because the artery is the largest and deepest of the three; is close to the femoral vein; and has no collateral circulation, so blood flow to the body area it supplies is compromised if complications occur

g. Regulation of arterial pressure involves neurohormonal control, which affects the volume of blood flow through the vessels and the elasticity of the resistance vessels

h. Seventy to ninety percent of coronary artery blood flow occurs during diastole

i. A mean arterial pressure (MAP) of at least 60 mm Hg is necessary to maintain autoregulation in the heart, brain, and kidneys

j. Systolic blood pressure (SBP) is the highest pressure occurring within the arterial system during a cardiac cycle; SBP determines the perfusion pressure on body tissues

k. Diastolic blood pressure (DBP) is the lowest pressure occurring within the arterial system during a cardiac cycle

l. MAP is the average pressure under which blood flows to the tissue during the cardiac cycle; it is calculated by the formula

$$MAP = \frac{SBP + 2DBP}{3}$$

m. Pulse pressure is the difference between SBP and DBP (normally 40 to 60 mm Hg) and reflects the vascular resistance of the arterial system and the stroke volume

2. Uses

a. Monitors direct intra-arterial pressures

b. Provides more accurate information about vascular capacity, blood volume, and heart pumping effectiveness

c. Allows routine blood specimens to be obtained from the line, which prevents the need for repeated needle sticks

3. Normal waveforms

a. A normal arterial waveform, noted by intra-arterial monitoring, consists of a rapid, sharp upstroke, a dicrotic notch, and a clear end-diastole; heart rate and rhythm may alter waveform configuration

b. The baseline of the wave is the aortic end-diastolic pressure (AEDP), which indicates the minimum pressure reached in the arteries during diastole

    c. The top of the wave is the peak systolic pressure (PSP), which indicates the maximum pressure reached in the arteries during systole; peak systolic pressure is heard as systolic blood pressure

    d. The dicrotic notch (DN) signifies the beginning of diastole

NORMAL ARTERIAL WAVEFORM

4. Implications of abnormal waveforms and readings

    a. For a patient in shock, SBP by cuff measurement is less than intra-arterial SBP; the difference may be greater in a patient with increased systemic vascular resistance caused by alpha-adrenergic stimulation, which may occur in a patient receiving vasopressors to increase blood pressure

    b. Intra-arterial SBP of less than 80 mm Hg, or 30 mm Hg less than the patient's normal SBP, indicates shock

    c. Intra-arterial SBP of greater than 150 mm Hg or a DBP greater than 100 mm Hg signifies hypertension

5. Patient care management

    a. Do not insert any medications (except heparin flush solution) through the intra-arterial line

    b. Level the air-fluid interface of the transducer at the catheter tip before obtaining readings

    c. Remove all air from the tubing and transducer because air bubbles dampen or distort the waveform

    d. Use a heparinized low-flow flush solution (1 to 2 units/ml) to maintain line patency and normal waveform transmission

    e. Calibrate the transducer to a known pressure to ensure accurate pressure readings; compare arterial line pressures to sphygmomanometer pressures at least once per shift; use correctly functioning intra-arterial line pressures, when possible, because they are more accurate than cuff pressures

    f. Keep in mind that a dampened waveform (as evidenced by loss of the dicrotic notch or a flattened upstroke) indicates air, blood, or clots in the arterial line

    g. Stabilize the catheter position with a dressing to prevent kinking

    h. Use Luer-Lok connectors to prevent breaks in the monitoring set-up

    i. Obtain routine blood specimens from the line

    j. Monitor for possible complications, such as infection, hemorrhage, decreased or absent pulses distal to the insertion site, embolus, or thrombus

    k. Check collateral circulation by performing Allen's test before inserting a catheter into the radial artery

    l. Keep in mind that brachial or femoral artery cannulation requires immobilization of the patient's affected arm, limiting his range of motion and self-care activities

    m. Remember that bleeding from femoral artery cannulation may be more difficult to control because of the difficulty in applying adequate pressure to the site, that large amounts of blood can be lost in the thigh before external signs of bleeding are evident, and that the site's proximity to the perineal area exposes it to bacterial contamination

C. Central venous pressure (CVP) monitoring

1. General information

    a. CVP is measured by a manometer connected to a central line or by a transducer connected to the proximal lumen of a pulmonary artery catheter; the catheter is located in the superior vena cava or the right atrium

    b. CVP is measured in millimeters of mercury (mm Hg) or centimeters of water (cm H_2O); to convert from one to another, use this equivalence: 1 mm Hg equals 1.36 cm H_2O

    c. CVP using a water manometer (most common) involves measuring the height of a column of water in a plastic or glass manometer with a three-way stopcock connected to a central line and attached to the I.V. tubing

    d. CVP represents the filling pressure or preload of the right ventricle or right ventricular end-diastolic pressure

    e. CVP can be used to assess fluid volume status because the venous bed contains 60% of blood volume

    f. CVP may be the last pressure to change in a patient with a rapidly changing cardiovascular status

    g. Trends in readings correlated to the patient's clinical condition provide more useful information about venous blood volume than does a single reading

2. Uses

    a. Evaluates right atrial and right ventricular pressure and function

    b. Monitors blood volume

    c. Assesses adequacy of central venous return

    d. Guides fluid volume administration by evaluating trends in the values obtained

    e. May differentiate right ventricular failure from left ventricular failure

3. Normal readings: 4 to 10 cm H_2O; 3 to 7 mm Hg

4. Implications of abnormal readings
   a. CVP is an unreliable indicator of left ventricular function
   b. CVP lower than 4 cm H_2O may indicate hypovolemia
   c. CVP higher than 10 cm H_2O may indicate hypervolemia or poor myocardial contractility
5. Patient care management
   a. Level the zero mark on the manometer to the phlebostatic axis for accuracy
   b. Indicate the level of the phlebostatic axis with an ink mark on the chest to ensure consistent readings
   c. Do not allow the manometer to overflow because this may cause contamination
   d. Observe for fluctuation of the fluid level with respiration; the level will drop with inspiration and rise with expiration from intrathoracic pressure changes
   e. Record pressures at the end of expiration after the fluid level stops fluctuating
   f. Observe for signs of common complications, such as infection and air embolism

D. Pulmonary artery pressure (PAP) monitoring
1. General information
   a. PAP is measured by a pulmonary artery (PA) catheter
   b. A PA catheter has a balloon tip, with two to five lumens or ports
   c. The catheter is passed through a large vein, such as the internal jugular or subclavian, into the right atrium of the heart
   d. After insertion, the catheter tip travels with the force of blood flow through the pulmonic valve, into the main PA or a primary branch, with the balloon deflated
   e. With the balloon inflated, the catheter "floats" out to occlude a smaller branch of the PA, allowing for measurement of pressure in front of the balloon; this pressure is called the pulmonary artery wedge pressure (PAWP), also known as the pulmonary capillary wedge pressure or pulmonary artery occlusive pressure
2. Uses
   a. Monitors direct intracardiac pressures
   b. Provides information about vascular capacity, blood volume, pump effectiveness, and tissue perfusion
   c. Indirectly reflects left ventricular end-diastolic pressure (LVEDP), which indicates left ventricular function
   d. The distal tip of the catheter measures PAP and PAWP; mixed venous blood specimens can be obtained from this port

PULMONARY ARTERY CATHETER

Pulmonary artery catheters are made of pliable, radiopaque, polyvinylchloride. This illustration shows a 110-cm (about 43¼") catheter, marked in 10-cm increments. It has distal and proximal lumens, which are fluid-filled for pressure monitoring; a thermistor lumen, which holds the wires connecting the thermistor to the cardiac output computer; a balloon inflation lumen with valve; and a pacemaker wire hub. As a result, this catheter can measure several pressures, as well as cardiac output.

Because catheters vary, depending on their manufacturer, consult the manufacturer's manual for additional details.

Thermistor hub
Connects to cardiac output computer to measure cardiac output.

Distal lumen hub
Attaches to pressure line to measure pulmonary artery pressure and pulmonary artery wedge pressure. I.V. flush solution exits from the distal port.

Balloon inflation valve
Receives the proper amount of gas (air or carbon dioxide) to inflate the balloon.

Proximal lumen hub
Attaches to pressure line to measure right atrial central venous pressure. To measure cardiac output, disconnect from pressure line and inject solution. I.V. flush solution or injectable solution exits from the proximal port.

Pacemaker wire hub
Allows for sequential electrical pacing.

Distal lumen port
Rests in the pulmonary artery.

Thermistor lumen
Detects blood temperature changes used to measure cardiac output. Located about 1½" (3.8 cm) from the catheter tip.

Balloon
Expands around catheter, when inflated, without occluding distal port.

Proximal lumen port
Rests in right atrium.

   e. The proximal port is used for continuous infusion of fluids or medications; it measures right atrial pressure with a stopcock configuration when the distal tip is in the PA

 3. Normal readings and waveforms: each pressure has a characteristic waveform
   a. Mean right atrial pressure: 3 to 6 mm Hg
   b. PAP: systolic, 17 to 32 mm Hg; diastolic, 4 to 13 mm Hg; mean, 9 to 19 mm Hg
   c. PAWP: 8 to 12 mm Hg

PULMONARY ARTERY CATHETER WAVEFORMS

RIGHT ATRIAL PRESSURE	RIGHT VENTRICULAR PRESSURE	PULMONARY ARTERY PRESSURE	PULMONARY ARTERY WEDGE PRESSURE
Normal range			
Mean: 3 to 6 mm Hg When the tip of the pulmonary artery catheter reaches the right atrium from the superior vena cava, the waveform on the oscilloscope screen or readout strip will look like this. When it does, the doctor will inflate the catheter's balloon, which will float the tip through the tricuspid valve and into the right ventricle.	Systolic: 17 to 32 mm Hg Diastolic: 1 to 7 mm Hg When the catheter tip reaches the patient's right ventricle, the waveform will look like this.	Systolic: 17 to 32 mm Hg Diastolic: 4 to 13 mm Hg Mean: 9 to 19 mm Hg A waveform like this indicates that the balloon has floated the catheter tip through the pulmonic valve into the pulmonary artery.	Mean: 8 to 12 mm Hg Blood flow in the pulmonary artery will then carry the catheter balloon into one of the pulmonary artery's many smaller branches. When the vessel becomes too narrow for the balloon to pass through, the balloon wedges in the vessel, occluding it. The monitor will then display a pulmonary artery wedge pressure waveform like this one.

4. Implications of abnormal readings
   a. In the absence of mitral disease, the mean PAWP closely approximates the LVEDP, because the mitral valve is open during diastole and pressure in the left atrium is equal to pressure in the left ventricle.
   b. The LVEDP correlates with the ventricular volume; variations in the PAWP indicate the earliest changes in left ventricular filling and function
   c. The PA diastolic pressure is normally 1 to 4 mm Hg higher than the PAWP; in the absence of lung disease, this pressure can be used to evaluate the left ventricular function
   d. PAWP cannot be greater than PA diastolic pressure, because of the pressure gradient within the heart and lungs

5. Patient care management
   a. Read pressures at the end of expiration because intrathoracic pressure changes from breathing, mechanical ventilation, or positive end-expiratory pressure will alter PAP and PAWP
   b. Keep in mind that right ventricular pressure readings (normal systolic is 17 to 32 mm Hg; normal diastolic is 1 to 7 mm Hg) are obtained only during catheter insertion
   c. Level the air-fluid interface of the transducer at the phlebostatic axis before obtaining readings, because an inverse change of 3 to 5 mm Hg is obtained for every inch of deviation from the established axis
   d. Remove all air from the tubing and transducer while setting up and monitoring, because air bubbles dampen or distort the waveform
   e. Use a heparinized low-flow flush solution (1 to 2 units/ml) to maintain line patency and normal waveform transmission
   f. Calibrate the transducer to a known pressure to ensure accurate pressure readings
   g. Stabilize the catheter position with a dressing to prevent kinking, to increase accuracy of the readings, and to minimize accidental dose fluctuations
   h. Inflate the balloon slowly while observing waveforms only to the point that occlusion (wedge) is obtained (do not exceed maximum balloon volume), to prevent overwedging and possible pulmonary infarction
   i. Do not aspirate the air from an inflated balloon; remove the syringe and allow the balloon to deflate passively to prevent possible balloon rupture
   j. Keep the balloon inflated no longer than absolutely necessary (less than 15 seconds) to prevent overwedging and possible pulmonary infarction
   k. Read the PAP and PAWP directly from hard copy or from a calibrated oscilloscope, because digital readouts are not reliable and do not reflect the end of expiration (pressures are averaged and updated digitally every 4 seconds)
   l. Avoid obtaining routine blood specimens from the catheter to decrease the risk of clotting and to ensure line patency
   m. Recognize that the patient is electrically sensitive with the catheter in place; a catheter entering the heart increases the risk of microshock, possibly producing ventricular fibrillation
   n. Monitor for possible complications, such as dysrhythmias, infection, air embolus, pneumothorax, or catheter clotting or kinking
   o. Notify the doctor if displayed waveforms show a permanent PAWP reading, right ventricular pressure tracing, or PAWP outside the given parameters

E. Cardiac output (CO) determination
   1. General information
      a. CO is the amount of blood the heart pumps per minute and is the product of the heart rate multiplied by stroke volume
      b. Serial CO determinations provide valuable information about left ventricular function

    c. The most common method used in a critical care area to measure CO is the thermodilution method, using the thermistor hub of the PA catheter

    d. Thermodilution is based on this principle: if a known amount of solution, at a known temperature, is injected into the bloodstream, the speed at which the solution moves can be reported as a temperature change downstream; the speed of this temperature change is calculated as CO by a cardiac output computer connected to the thermistor hub port of the PA catheter

    e. Iced injectate or room temperature injectate can be used; a computation constant set on the cardiac output computer can be changed to accommodate variations in temperature, volume, and catheter size

    f. Advantages include rapid, reliable results unaffected by O_2; no need to withdraw blood; and only one person needed to perform the procedure

    g. Disadvantages include inaccuracy with low CO and with mitral or tricuspid insufficiency or shunts; procedure may pose an electrical hazard

    h. Because CO varies among individuals, the cardiac index (CI) standardizes the CO results; patients with different body sizes can be compared. CI is calculated by dividing the CO by the body surface area (obtained from a standard chart) to adjust for body size

    i. CI is a more precise measurement than CO and is more commonly used to evaluate the patient's status

2. Uses

    a. Assesses left ventricular function

    b. Evaluates the adequacy of CO to help determine the extent of oxygen delivery to the tissues

    c. Assesses the patient's response to therapy

3. Normal readings

    a. CO: 4 to 8 liters/minute

    b. CI: 2.5 to 4.3 liters/minute/m²

4. Implications of abnormal readings

    a. CI less than 2.2 liters/minute/m² indicates hypoperfusion to the tissues

    b. CI less than 1.8 liters/minute/m² suggests cardiogenic shock

    c. CI greater than 4.3 liters/minute/m² may be found in the early stages of septic shock or in situations in which the heart is compensating for increased metabolic demands (thyrotoxicosis, fever, exercise, and certain tumors)

5. Patient care management

    a. Measure the volume of injectate exactly to ensure accurate results

    b. Ensure that the computation constant is set at the correct number for volume and temperature of injectate

    c. Monitor the injectate's temperature carefully so that the computer can correctly calculate any temperature change

    d. Ensure representative CO measurements by taking three measurements and averaging the results; measurements should be within 10% of each other, and any readings outside this range should not be counted

    e. Inject the solution at end-expiration to negate the effects of intrathoracic pressure

  f. Cover the electrical port of the PA catheter with the cap when the computer cable is disconnected, to reduce the risk of microshock

F. Mixed venous oxygen saturation (SVO$_2$) measurements
 1. General information
  a. Continuous mixed SVO$_2$ assesses the balance between oxygen supply and tissue demand for oxygen; it reflects the body's ability to meet tissue oxygen needs
  b. A fiberoptic PA catheter is used to measure the average percentage of oxygen bound to hemoglobin in venous blood
  c. Its measurement indicates overall tissue oxygen and is recorded by an oximeter
  d. An oximeter produces a digital readout of SVO$_2$, along with a strip recorder, to provide a permanent written record
  e. SVO$_2$ is influenced by two primary factors: oxygen transport and tissue oxygen consumption
  f. A change in one or both of these triggers compensation, producing changes in the SVO$_2$ level
 2. Uses
  a. Aids in diagnosis and treatment of a critical care patient with a life-threatening condition, such as shock
  b. Can serve as an early guide to intervention because changes in SVO$_2$ values reflect changes in oxygen demand or delivery
  c. May reduce repetitive arterial blood sampling, which can contribute to significant blood loss and cost
 3. Normal readings: normal mixed SVO$_2$ is 60% to 80%
 4. Implications of abnormal readings
  a. Changes in venous oxygen pressure—even in small amounts—produce large changes in SVO$_2$
  b. Decreased SVO$_2$ reflects problems associated with increased oxygen demands or decreased oxygen delivery caused by a decrease in hemoglobin, arterial oxygen saturation, or CO
  c. Decreased SVO$_2$ can occur in a patient with anemia, hyperthermia, seizures, fever, shivering, dysrhythmias, or heart failure
  d. Increased SVO$_2$ reflects problems associated with increased oxygen delivery, artifact, decreased oxygen uptake, and increased CO
  e. Increased SVO$_2$ can occur in a patient with polycythemia, anesthesia, hypothermia, left-to-right shunt, inotropic drug administration, increased fraction of inspired oxygen from mechanical ventilation, or septic shock
 5. Patient care management
  a. Evaluate the effects of nursing interventions (such as suctioning, personal care activities, changes in oxygen therapy delivery, and drug administration) on SVO$_2$ readings
  b. Recognize that complications related to SVO$_2$ monitoring are associated with PAP monitoring
  c. See "Patient care management," item D.5, in this section for other considerations

Points to Remember

Frequency of hemodynamic measurements is determined by the patient's clinical condition.

Pressure values obtained should be assessed in relation to the patient's baseline hemodynamic pressure and should be viewed as trends.

Actions based on data obtained by hemodynamic monitoring should be supported by other assessment findings.

The clinical reliability of hemodynamic readings is directly related to the consistency and accuracy of the interpreter's measurements.

Glossary

Calibration—application of a known quantity of pressure to the transducer; the accuracy of the pressure measurement displayed can be evaluated with a built-in mechanism on the monitor or with a fluid-filled or mercury manometer

Left ventricular end-diastolic pressure (LVEDP)—pressure in the left ventricle at the end of diastole just before systolic contraction; it closely approximates the mean pulmonary arterial wedge pressure in the absence of mitral valve disease

Phlebostatic axis—imaginary line, drawn at the fourth intercostal space mid-axillary line, that serves as the reference point for the right atrium

Transducer—device that converts the pressure transmitted by the fluid-filled tubing into an electrical signal represented by waveforms on an oscilloscope

Zero reference point—point where air and fluid meet; physiologic pressures are relative to atmospheric pressure, so transducers must be balanced ("zeroed") at atmospheric pressure

Intracranial Pressure Monitoring

Learning Objectives

After studying this section, the reader should be able to:

- Identify the basic principles of intracranial pressure (ICP) monitoring.

- Describe advantages and disadvantages for each method of ICP monitoring.

- List the general information obtained through ICP monitoring.

- Describe care management for the patient being monitored for ICP.

IX. Intracranial Pressure Monitoring

A. **Basic concepts**
1. ICP is monitored by using a sensor or catheter inserted into a specific cranial area
2. The three cranial areas monitored most frequently are the lateral ventricle, the subarachnoid space, and the epidural space; epidural monitoring has limited usefulness, so it is used infrequently in major trauma centers
3. ICP monitoring has specific requirements
    a. It requires an informed consent
    b. Aseptic technique is essential during the insertion and maintenance of the monitoring device
    c. The system must always be free of air to reproduce intracranial waveforms accurately; a continuous-flush device is contraindicated
    d. The transducer is leveled to the foramen of Monro
    e. The monitor must be balanced and calibrated routinely, according to institutional policy
    f. Variations in values should be regarded as trends
4. ICP is determined by the components within the cranial vault
    a. Brain tissue volume
    b. Cerebrospinal fluid (CSF)
    c. Blood volume
5. ICPs are dynamic
    a. They vary with arterial pulsations, respirations, and such activities as coughing and sneezing
    b. The Monro-Kellie hypothesis states that when the volume of one component increases, the total pressure will increase unless a reciprocal change is made in another component
6. Compensation for increased ICP occurs through:
    a. Displacement of CSF (most compensation occurs this way)
    b. Reduction of cerebral blood volume
    c. Displacement of brain tissue (herniation)
7. Systemic arterial pressure and ICP affect cerebral perfusion
    a. Cerebral perfusion pressure (CPP) provides an estimate of cerebral blood flow
    b. CPP, the difference between cerebral arterial and venous pressure, is calculated by the formula CPP = mean arterial pressure (MAP) − ICP
    c. As the formula indicates, CPP can be affected by changes in MAP or ICP
    d. Normal cerebral blood flow is maintained with CPP by autoregulatory factors in a range of 40 to 130 mm Hg
    e. If CPP falls outside this range, blood flow to the brain is impaired

8. Uses
   a. Helps prevent or minimize neurologic damage in a patient with neurologic problems, such as head trauma (especially closed head injuries), ruptured cerebral aneurysms, Reye's syndrome, known or suspected hydrocephalus, or brain tumor
   b. Allows for observation of trends and changes in the patient's condition
   c. Indicates a change in ICP dynamics before other signs are clinically present
9. Patient care management varies with the monitoring method; for a patient with a ventricular catheter or subarachnoid screw:
   a. Analyze pressure data for trends, which are more significant than any specific reading
   b. Monitor CPP by the formula CPP = MAP − ICP
   c. Assess for abnormal waveforms: A (plateau), B, or C waves; report A waves to the doctor because these are clinically significant
   d. Maintain the transducer at the foramen of Monro (the external landmark is the outer canthus of the eye or the top of the ear) to ensure accurate readings
   e. Maintain a fluid-filled pressure system; do not connect the monitoring device to a pressure bag or a continuous-infusion system
   f. If the waveforms are decreased or dampened, flush the system only if institutional policy allows (do not aspirate the system to attempt to remove the obstruction)
   g. Zero and calibrate the transducer with changes in readings according to institutional policy
   h. Maintain aseptic technique during insertion and maintenance to minimize the risk of infection
   i. Check the system for leaks; use Luer-Lok connectors when possible
   j. Change the transducer, tubing, and dressing according to institutional policy

B. Normal and abnormal readings
1. Normal readings
   a. ICP ranges from 0 to 10 mm Hg, with an upper limit of 15 mm Hg
   b. CPP is 80 to 90 mm Hg
   c. Waveform appearance depends on the measurement method and associated pathology and can be affected by arterial pulsation, cerebral vasodilation, and changes in venous outflow; may resemble arterial pressure or central venous pressure waveforms
2. Implications of abnormal readings
   a. If MAP decreases or ICP increases, CPP decreases
   b. If CPP decreases below 60 mm Hg, ischemia occurs within the brain
   c. If MAP equals ICP, blood flow ceases within the brain

    d. Waveform variations, known as A, B, or C waves, may occur

    e. *A waves* (plateau waves) are rapid, spontaneous, sustained increases in pressure, usually from 50 to 100 mm Hg but sometimes approaching 200 mm Hg, that last 5 to 20 minutes before falling spontaneously; the waves indicate intracranial decompensation and compression

    f. *B waves* are sharp, small waves with pressure up to 50 mm Hg; they correspond to changes in respiration and may be caused by variations in cerebral blood volume

    g. *C waves* are small, rhythmic waves with pressures up to 20 mm Hg that occur at a rate of up to 6/minute; they are related to pressure and, like A waves, indicate intracranial compression

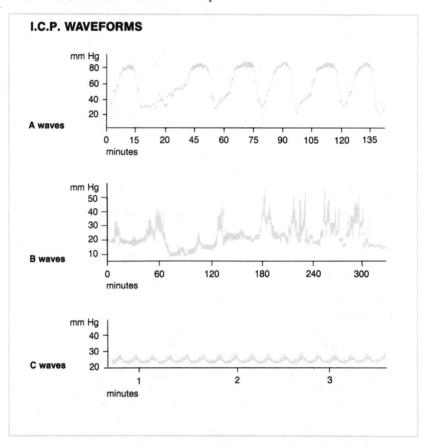

C. Intraventricular ICP monitoring

1. General information
    a. The ventricular catheter usually is inserted via a drill hole through the dura into the anterior horn of the lateral ventricle in the nondominant hemisphere
    b. The catheter is sometimes inserted into the posterior horn of the lateral ventricle in the nondominant hemisphere
    c. The procedure is performed with the patient under a local anesthetic
    d. The catheter is connected to a pressure transducer by a stopcock or by pressure tubing
2. Advantages
    a. Measures CSF pressure directly (most accurate method)
    b. Therapeutically drains excess CSF
    c. Allows for recalibration of the transducer
    d. Offers the ability to test intracranial volume pressure responses (a measure of intracranial elastance and compliance)
    e. Allows instillation of contrast media for testing
3. Disadvantages
    a. Requires puncturing of the brain, increasing the risk of brain tissue damage
    b. Increases risk of intracranial infection
    c. Makes insertion difficult if the ventricles are small or displaced
    d. May cause excess loss of CSF
    e. May permit blood clots to block catheter

D. Subarachnoid screw monitoring

1. General information
    a. A hollow screw is inserted via a burr hole through the skull into the subarachnoid space
    b. The procedure is performed with the patient under a local anesthetic
    c. The catheter is connected to a pressure transducer by a stopcock or by pressure tubing
2. Advantages
    a. Measures CSF pressure directly
    b. Therapeutically drains CSF
    c. Allows for recalibration of the transducer
3. Disadvantages
    a. Increases risk of intracranial infection
    b. May cause excess loss of CSF
    c. Does not allow instillation of contrast media
    d. May be blocked by swelling brain tissue

E. Epidural monitoring
  1. General information
      a. An intracranial transducer or balloon is inserted between the skull and dura
      b. The transducer or balloon is connected to an external monitor
  2. Advantages
      a. Poses less danger of infection than other methods
      b. Monitors ICP without opening dura
  3. Disadvantages
      a. May not accurately reflect ICP because epidural pressure is higher than intraventricular pressure
      b. Does not allow for draining of CSF
      c. Increases the possibility of inaccurate readings because some systems cannot be recalibrated
      d. Does not allow for testing of volume pressure responses (a measure of intracranial elastance and compliance)

Points to Remember

Intracranial pressure is dynamic and is affected by most activities of daily living.

Systemic arterial pressure and intracranial pressure affect cerebral perfusion.

The trend in data is more significant than any one reading.

The most accurate method of ICP monitoring is the intraventricular method.

Glossary

Epidural space—space surrounding the dura mater directly below the skull

Foramen of Monro—passage between the lateral and third ventricles within the brain; used as an internal landmark for leveling the ICP monitor transducer

Herniation of the brain—protrusion of part of the brain through an abnormal opening

Volume pressure response—test for intracranial elastance and compliance, performed by a doctor; sterile saline solution is injected into the intraventricular catheter or subarachnoid screw, and changes in pressure readings are recorded to assess altered compensation

Continuous Cardiac Monitoring

Learning Objectives

After studying this section, the reader should be able to:

- Describe the general principles for the patient requiring continuous cardiac monitoring.

- Identify the common leads used for cardiac monitoring.

- Discuss care management for a patient undergoing cardiac monitoring.

- Explain what is represented by the normal electrocardiographic (ECG) waveforms, segments, and intervals.

- Identify the ECG characteristics of normal sinus rhythm.

X. Continuous Cardiac Monitoring

A. Basic concepts

1. Cardiac monitoring measures the heart's electrical activity, displayed as waveforms, by the placement of electrodes on the chest
   a. Each waveform represents a particular event in the cardiac cycle
   b. Waveforms are identified by the letters P, Q, R, S, and T
2. Heart rate, rhythm, and conduction are displayed continuously on a monitor screen
3. The patient may be monitored continuously while in bed (known as hardwire monitoring) or while ambulatory (known as telemetry)
   a. Electrodes are placed on the chest to allow for patient mobility; they are not placed on bony prominences
   b. The conductant used on the electrodes must be moist
4. Monitoring equipment varies, but most have basic components:
   a. Oscilloscope—a screen that displays the ECG tracing; most tracings can be frozen to stop the movement
   b. Alarms—controls that permit the user to set limits for fast or slow heart rates
   c. Hard copy—a printout of the ECG tracing on standardized graph paper
5. Rate and rhythm determination may be made from the monitor or hard copy
   a. Time is measured along the horizontal axis on the hard copy; each small block represents 0.04 second, and each large block represents 0.20 second
   b. The hard copy is usually marked at 3- to 6-second intervals
   c. The recording speed on the monitor and hard copy should be set at 25 mm/second so that 300 large blocks pass through the recorder each minute
   d. The rate may be obtained from a digital readout display or calculated from the hard copy by determining the number of cardiac cycles in a 6-second interval and multiplying by 10
   e. The rhythm may be determined on the hard copy by measuring the length between the R-R intervals (determines ventricular rhythm) or P-P intervals (determines atrial rhythm) using calipers; the rhythm is regular if the lengths of the shortest and longest intervals measured differ by less than 0.16 second
6. Continuous monitoring is used to:
   a. Monitor cardiac function in critically ill patients
   b. Observe symptomatic dysrhythmia or cardiac pathology
   c. Evaluate drug, fluid, or electrolyte therapy
7. Cardiac monitoring limitations
   a. Measures only electrical activity
   b. Is not an indicator of cardiac mechanical function
   c. Must be correlated with the patient's clinical status
   d. Is not a substitute for a 12-lead diagnostic ECG

8. Patient care management
    a. Explain the procedure to the patient
    b. Prepare the skin for electrode placement by shaving, cleansing, and abrading to decrease skin resistance to the transmission of electrical signals from the heart
    c. Place the electrodes in the correct locations based on lead type
    d. Prevent artifact or possible electrical shock by properly grounding the equipment
    e. Set the high- and low-rate alarms
    f. Observe the monitor for changes in rate, rhythm, or conduction; document and report significant changes to the doctor
    g. Document episodes of chest pain or diaphoresis, and report these to the doctor, especially if they occur concurrently with monitor changes

B. **Types of leads**
    1. Two common types of monitoring leads are lead II and MCL_1; waveform deflection is determined by the lead selection
    2. Lead II produces *upright* waveform deflections; P waves are seen clearly
        a. The (+) electrode is placed at the left midclavicular line, at or below the fifth intercostal space
        b. The (−) electrode is placed on the right shoulder, below the clavicle
        c. The ground electrode stabilizes the electrical pattern and may be placed at any location on the body
    3. MCL_1 produces *inverted* waveform deflections; it simulates the precordial V_1 lead of a 12-lead ECG and offers more diagnostic advantages for identifying ectopy and blocks
        a. The (+) electrode is placed at the fourth intercostal space, on the right sternal border
        b. The (−) electrode is placed on the left shoulder, below the clavicle
        c. The ground electrode stabilizes the electrical pattern and may be placed at any location on the body

C. **Characteristics of a normal cardiac cycle**
    1. The P wave represents atrial depolarization and indicates sinoatrial (SA) node function
        a. Location: precedes the QRS complex
        b. Duration: 0.06 to 0.11 second
        c. Configuration: usually symmetrically rounded and upright in lead II; may be diphasic (positive and negative), flat, or inverted in MCL_1
    2. The QRS complex represents ventricular depolarization
        a. Location: follows the PR interval
        b. Duration: less than 0.10 second
        c. Configuration: different in each lead; the Q wave is the first negative deflection (may not always appear); the R wave is the first positive deflection; the S wave is the negative deflection after the R wave

3. The T wave represents ventricular repolarization
   a. Location: follows the S wave and ST segment
   b. Duration: not usually measured
   c. Configuration: usually rounded, upright, smooth, and less than 5 mm in lead II; direction of deflection in MCL_1 is variable
4. The PR interval represents the time it takes the impulse to reach the Purkinje fibers
   a. Location: extends from beginning of P wave to beginning of QRS complex
   b. Duration: 0.12 to 0.20 second
5. The ST segment represents the end of ventricular depolarization and the beginning of repolarization
   a. Location: extends from end of S wave to beginning of T wave
   b. Duration: not usually measured
   c. Configuration: usually isoelectric, not varying more than 1 mm (one small vertical block)

NORMAL CARDIAC CYCLE

D. Normal readings: Normal sinus rhythm
   1. Definition: rhythm originating in the sinus node with all characteristics being normal; indicates lack of cardiac disease and requires no intervention
   2. ECG characteristics
      a. Rate: 60 to 100 beats/minute
      b. Rhythm: regular; atrial and ventricular are the same
      c. P wave: usually rounded and upright and lasting 0.06 to 0.11 second
      d. PR interval: 0.12 to 0.20 second
      e. QRS complex: no longer than 0.10 second
      f. ST segment: flat
      g. T wave: usually upright, rounded, and smooth

Points to Remember

Cardiac monitoring transforms the heart's electrical activity into a series of waveforms.

Cardiac monitoring measures only cardiac electrical activity and is not an indicator of cardiac mechanical function.

Each cardiac monitoring lead generates its own characteristic waveforms.

The basic waveforms are the P wave, the QRS complex, and the T wave.

Glossary

Calipers—two-legged instrument used to measure distance and determine rhythm on a cardiac monitoring strip

Isoelectric—showing no variation in electric potential (refers to the flat line between each waveform on the hard copy)

Lead—graphic illustration of the electrical potential difference between two points on the skin surface

Oscilloscope—screen that displays the ECG tracing

Telemetry—means of continuous cardiac monitoring for an ambulatory patient, using a battery-powered generator that transmits the signal to a central stationary monitor screen

Cardiac Dysrhythmias

Learning Objectives

After studying this section, the reader should be able to:

- Discuss general principles of dysrhythmia interpretation.

- Describe the ECG characteristics for each type of dysrhythmia.

- Identify life-threatening dysrhythmias.

- Describe care management for the patient with a life-threatening dysrhythmia.

XI. Cardiac Dysrhythmias

A. Basic concepts
1. Dysrhythmia is any disturbance in the normal rhythm of the heartbeat
2. Disturbances or irregularities in rhythm occur because of three mechanisms:
    a. Alteration in automaticity
    b. Alteration in conductivity
    c. Alteration in automaticity and conductivity
3. Five steps are used to interpret dysrhythmias
    a. Determine the rate (both atrial and ventricular)
    b. Determine the rhythm (regular or irregular)
    c. Analyze the P waves (normal, with one for each QRS)
    d. Measure the PR interval (intervals outside the normal range indicate a conduction disturbance)
    e. Measure the duration of the QRS complex (a duration longer than normal indicates a ventricular conduction disturbance)
4. Dysrhythmia interpretation may require analysis of the rhythm in more than one lead
5. Dysrhythmias are classified according to site:
    a. Sinus
    b. Atrial
    c. Junctional
    d. Ventricular
    e. Atrioventricular (AV)

B. Sinus bradycardia
1. Definition: dysrhythmia in which all impulses originate in the sinus node, but the rate is less than 60 beats/minute
2. ECG characteristics
    a. Rate: less than 60 beats/minute for atrial and ventricular rates
    b. Rhythm: regular; atrial and ventricular are the same
    c. P wave: normal
    d. PR interval: within normal limits
    e. QRS complex: within normal limits
    f. ST segment: normal
    g. T wave: normal
3. Possible causes
    a. Exercise or sleep (may be normal)
    b. Increased intracranial pressure
    c. Increased vagal tone from straining or vomiting
    d. Mechanical ventilation
    e. Sick sinus syndrome
    f. Hypothyroidism
    g. Hyperkalemia
    h. Drug therapy with beta blockers or sympatholytics

4. Clinical significance depends on the cause and symptoms
5. Patient care management
   a. Do not intervene if the patient is asymptomatic
   b. Treat the underlying cause

C. Sinus tachycardia

1. Definition: dysrhythmia in which all impulses originate in the sinus node, but the rate is accelerated
2. ECG characteristics
   a. Rate: atrial and ventricular rates 100 to 160 beats/minute
   b. Rhythm: regular; atrial and ventricular are the same
   c. P wave: normal but may not be visible if the rate exceeds 140 beats/minute
   d. PR interval: within normal limits
   e. QRS complex: within normal limits
   f. ST segment: normal
   g. T wave: normal
3. Possible causes
   a. Normal physiologic response to the demand for increased oxygen during stress or activity
   b. Caffeine, nicotine, or alcohol
   c. Such drugs as adrenergics, anticholinergics, and some antiarrhythmics
   d. Digitalis toxicity
   e. Decrease in vagal tone and increase in sympathetic tone
   f. Hyperthyroidism
   g. Anemia, hypovolemia, or hypertension
4. Clinical significance
   a. None if it is a normal response
   b. Increased rate increases myocardial oxygen demand and can lead to ischemia and myocardial damage
5. Patient care management
   a. Treat the underlying cause
   b. Observe the patient for signs and symptoms of hypoxia and congestive heart failure
   c. Apply vagal stimulation, such as Valsalva's maneuver or carotid sinus massage

D. Atrial fibrillation

1. Definition: 400 to 500 unorganized ectopic impulses/minute in the atria, producing atrial quiver instead of contraction
2. ECG characteristics
   a. Rate: atrial rate is indiscernible; ventricular rate is usually 100 to 150 beats/minute
   b. Rhythm: atrial and ventricular grossly irregular

    c. P wave: none
    d. PR interval: indiscernible
    e. QRS complex: within normal limits
    f. ST segment: not identifiable
    g. T wave: not identifiable
  3. Possible causes
    a. Valvular disease
    b. Coronary artery disease (CAD)
    c. Cardiomyopathy
    d. Myocardial infarction (MI)
    e. Constrictive pericarditis
    f. Congestive heart failure (CHF)
    g. Chronic obstructive pulmonary disease (COPD)
    h. Thyrotoxicosis
    i. Increased sympathetic activity
  4. Clinical significance
    a. Cardiac output may be decreased by as much as 30%
    b. Mural thrombi may develop in the atria and migrate to the pulmonary or systemic circulation, causing a pulmonary or peripheral embolus
  5. Patient care management
    a. Administer digitalis, verapamil, or beta blockers to increase AV node refractoriness, or quinidine or procainamide to prolong atrial refractoriness
    b. Initiate Valsalva's maneuver or carotid sinus massage, which may reduce the rapid ventricular rate if it is not chronic atrial fibrillation
    c. Administer anticoagulants to decrease clot formation
    d. Deliver synchronized cardioversion if the patient is hemodynamically unstable
    e. Treat the underlying cause to prevent recurrence

E. Atrial flutter

  1. Definition: dysrhythmia characterized by a rapid atrial rate of 250 to 350 beats/minute
  2. ECG characteristics
    a. Rate: atrial rate may be 250 to 350 beats/minute; ventricular rate depends on degree of AV block, usually 60 to 100 beats/minute; the ratio of atrial to ventricular conduction may be 1:2, 1:3, or 1:4
    b. Rhythm: atrial and ventricular are usually regular
    c. P wave: saw-toothed, flutter waves; two, three, or four for each QRS complex
    d. PR interval: not measurable
    e. QRS complex: usually within normal limits
    f. ST segment: not identifiable
    g. T wave: not identifiable

3. Possible causes
   a. MI
   b. Valvular disease
   c. Cor pulmonale
   d. Pericarditis
   e. Digitalis toxicity
   f. Hyperthyroidism
   g. Pulmonary embolism
   h. Postoperative revascularization
4. Clinical significance
   a. Depends on the ventricular rate
   b. More difficult to convert than atrial fibrillation
5. Patient care management
   a. Administer verapamil, digitalis (unless the condition is caused by digitalis toxicity), or propranolol
   b. Administer quinidine, which may convert flutter to fibrillation
   c. Deliver synchronized cardioversion if the ventricular rate is rapid

F. **First-degree AV block**
   1. Definition: conduction disturbance in which the electrical impulses are delayed at the AV node
   2. ECG characteristics
      a. Rate: Atrial and ventricular rates 60 to 100 beats/minute
      b. Rhythm: atrial and ventricular regular
      c. P wave: normal
      d. PR interval: prolonged more than 0.20 second but constant
      e. QRS complex: usually within normal limits
      f. ST segment: normal
      g. T wave: normal
   3. Possible causes
      a. Such drugs as quinidine, procainamide, digitalis, or propranolol
      b. Rheumatic fever
      c. Chronic degeneration of the conduction system
      d. Potassium imbalance
      e. Myocardial ischemia or infarction
      f. Hypothyroidism
   4. Clinical significance: none
   5. Patient care management
      a. Monitor carefully for AV block progressing to higher degree
      b. Withhold any drug that may be the cause
      c. Do not intervene if the patient is asymptomatic

G. **Second-degree AV block, Mobitz Type I**
   1. Definition: conduction disturbance in which the AV node conducts each successive impulse earlier and earlier, until an impulse arrives during the absolute refractory period and cannot be conducted

2. ECG characteristics
   a. Rate: atrial rate is greater than ventricular, but both are usually within normal limits
   b. Rhythm: atrial is regular; ventricular is irregular because of progressive shortening of the R-R interval
   c. P wave: normal
   d. PR interval: progressively lengthens with each cycle until a P wave appears without a QRS complex
   e. QRS complex: normal, but is dropped periodically
   f. ST segment: within normal limits
   g. T wave: normal
3. Possible causes
   a. Inferior wall MI
   b. Digitalis toxicity
   c. Acute rheumatic fever
   d. Electrolyte imbalance
   e. Drug therapy with quinidine or procainamide
4. Clinical significance
   a. Prognosis is good if the patient is asymptomatic
   b. Second-degree AV block may progress to a more serious block
5. Patient care management
   a. Treat the underlying cause
   b. Use atropine or prepare the symptomatic patient for insertion of a temporary pacemaker

H. Second-degree AV block, Mobitz Type II
1. Definition: conduction disturbance in which dropped beats occur without warning, because the abnormality is in the Bundle of His or the bundle branches
2. ECG characteristics
   a. Rate: atrial is usually within normal limits; ventricular is slower
   b. Rhythm: atrial is regular; ventricular may be irregular
   c. P wave: normal
   d. PR interval: within normal limits or prolonged, but always constant
   e. QRS complex: normal, but periodically absent
   f. ST segment: normal unless myocardial ischemia or damage is present
   g. T wave: normal
3. Possible causes
   a. Anterior wall MI
   b. Severe CAD
   c. Other organic heart disease
4. Clinical significance
   a. More serious than Mobitz Type I because it is unpredictable
   b. May progress to third-degree (complete) heart block

5. Patient care management
   a. Administer vasoactive drugs to maintain blood pressure and cardiac output
   b. Prepare the patient for insertion of a temporary pacemaker to stabilize hemodynamic status
   c. Prepare the patient for insertion of a permanent pacemaker to prevent ventricular standstill

I. **Third-degree AV block (complete heart block)**
   1. Definition: condition in which all atrial impulses are blocked at the AV junction and a secondary pacemaker (in the junction or ventricle) stimulates the ventricles; the atria and ventricles beat independently
   2. ECG characteristics
      a. Rate: atrial is faster than ventricular, which is usually less than 45 beats/minute
      b. Rhythm: atrial has regular P-P intervals and ventricular has regular R-R intervals, but no relationship exists between the atrial and ventricular rhythm
      c. P wave: normal
      d. PR interval: not applicable because the atria and ventricles beat independently of each other; may appear to vary
      e. QRS complex: configuration depends on where the ventricular stimulus originates; may be narrow, wide, or bizarre
      f. ST segment: normal
      g. T wave: normal
   3. Possible causes
      a. Anterior wall MI
      b. Acute digitalis toxicity
      c. Postoperative complication of mitral or aortic valve replacement
      d. Rheumatic fever
      e. Congenital abnormalities
   4. Clinical significance
      a. Slow ventricular rates decrease cardiac output
      b. Ventricular dysrhythmias may develop if a secondary pacemaker in the ventricle becomes irritable
      c. Failure of a ventricular pacemaker results in cardiac arrest
   5. Patient care management
      a. Administer vasoactive drugs to maintain blood pressure and cardiac output
      b. Prepare the patient for insertion of a temporary pacemaker to stabilize hemodynamic status
      c. Prepare the patient for insertion of a permanent pacemaker to prevent ventricular standstill

J. Left bundle-branch block (LBBB)

1. Definition: conduction delay in the left posterior and anterior branches of the left bundle that disrupts normal left-to-right ventricular activation; an incomplete LBBB represents an altered conduction in either the posterior or the anterior branch

2. ECG characteristics
    a. Rate: atrial and ventricular within normal limits
    b. Rhythm: atrial and ventricular regular
    c. P wave: normal
    d. PR interval: within normal limits
    e. QRS complex: complete LBBB shows duration of 0.12 second or greater; incomplete LBBB shows duration between 0.10 and 0.12 second (deflection of the QRS complex varies with lead selection)
    f. ST segment: usually abnormal in size and configuration and occurring in opposite direction of QRS complex
    g. T wave: deflection is in opposite direction of QRS complex in most leads

3. Possible causes
    a. MI
    b. Hypertension
    c. CAD
    d. Myocarditis
    e. Valvular disease
    f. Congenital abnormalities
    g. Ventricular hypertrophy
    h. Degenerative diseases of the cardiac conduction system

4. Clinical significance
    a. Usually does not occur in healthy people
    b. Indicates underlying heart disease
    c. LBBB with left axis deviation associated with higher morbidity and mortality

5. Patient care management
    a. Usually, none is required for the block itself
    b. Prepare the patient for insertion of a pacemaker (if it is required to treat LBBB with acute anteroseptal MI)
    c. Treat the underlying cause

K. Right bundle-branch block (RBBB)

1. Definition: conduction delay in the right bundle branch
    a. It causes the right ventricle to be activated late
    b. Depolarizing forces spread through the system from the left ventricle instead of almost simultaneously with the left ventricle

2. ECG characteristics
    a. Rate: atrial and ventricular within normal limits
    b. Rhythm: atrial and ventricular regular
    c. P wave: normal

    d. PR interval: within normal limits
    e. QRS complex: complete RBBB shows duration of 0.12 second or greater; incomplete RBBB shows duration between 0.10 and 0.12 second (deflection of the QRS complex varies with lead selection)
    f. ST segment: usually abnormal and opposite in direction to QRS complex
    g. T wave: deflection in opposite direction of QRS complex

3. Possible causes
    a. Acute heart failure
    b. CAD
    c. MI
    d. Hypokalemia
    e. Digitalis toxicity
    f. Valvular or congenital anomalies
    g. Right ventricular hypertrophy
    h. Acute pulmonary embolism
    i. Atherosclerosis of the conduction system
    j. Right heart catheterization

4. Clinical significance: aids in diagnosis of other conditions

5. Patient care management
    a. Usually, none is required for the block itself
    b. Prepare the patient for insertion of a pacemaker (if it is required to treat RBBB with acute anteroseptal MI)
    c. Treat the underlying cause

L. Junctional escape rhythm

1. Definition: supraventricular dysrhythmia originating in the AV junction that occurs as an escape or safety mechanism when the SA node's pacing ability fails

2. ECG characteristics
    a. Rate: atrial and ventricular rates 40 to 60 beats/minute
    b. Rhythm: atrial and ventricular regular
    c. P wave: may occur before or after the QRS complex or may be absent (hidden in the QRS)
    d. PR interval: varies, depending on location of the P wave
    e. QRS complex: within normal limits
    f. ST segment: normal
    g. T wave: normal

3. Possible causes
    a. Digitalis toxicity
    b. Inferior wall MI
    c. Hypoxia
    d. Vagal stimulation
    e. Rheumatic fever
    f. Valvular surgery

    4. Clinical significance
      a. Serious but not life-threatening
      b. Protects the heart from standstill
    5. Patient care management
      a. Administer atropine to increase the heart rate
      b. Prepare the patient for insertion of a temporary pacemaker
      c. Treat the underlying cause
      d. Do not treat an asymptomatic patient

M. Premature atrial contraction
    1. Definition: beat that originates outside the sinoatrial (SA) node, usually because of an irritable focus in the atria
    2. ECG characteristics
      a. Rate: atrial and ventricular usually within normal limits
      b. Rhythm: atrial and ventricular irregular because of the premature beat; underlying rhythm may be regular
      c. P wave: premature and abnormal in the premature beat
      d. PR interval: longer or shorter than normal in the premature beat
      e. QRS complex: usually within normal limits in the premature beat
      f. ST segment: normal
      g. T wave: normal or may be distorted if the P wave is early
    3. Possible causes
      a. CHF
      b. CAD
      c. Valvular heart disease
      d. COPD
      e. Hypoxia
      f. Stress
      g. Fatigue
      h. Caffeine, tobacco, or alcohol
    4. Clinical significance
      a. Rarely dangerous in the patient without heart disease
      b. May precipitate more serious dysrhythmia, such as atrial fibrillation or flutter
      c. May indicate CHF or electrolyte imbalance
    5. Patient care management
      a. Monitor for signs and symptoms of heart failure
      b. Administer drug therapy, which may include digitalis, verapamil, or quinidine
      c. Eliminate caffeine, tobacco, and alcohol

N. Premature junctional contraction
    1. Definition: contraction from a stimulus in the AV junctional tissue that paces the heart for a single beat prematurely
    2. ECG characteristics
      a. Rate: atrial and ventricular usually the same

    b. Rhythm: atrial and ventricular irregular; R-R interval shorter for the premature beat

    c. P wave: inverted or abnormally shaped in the premature beat; may occur before or after the QRS complex or may be absent (hidden in the QRS)

    d. PR interval: shorter than 0.12 second in the premature beat if the P wave occurs before the QRS complex

    e. QRS complex: occurs prematurely but is usually normal

    f. ST segment: may be distorted if the P wave occurs after the QRS complex

    g. T wave: normal unless the P wave occurs after the QRS complex

  3. Possible causes

    a. Digitalis toxicity

    b. Myocardial ischemia or infarction

    c. Excessive caffeine or amphetamine ingestion

  4. Clinical significance

    a. Usually harmless unless it occurs frequently; then it represents irritability that may precipitate a more dangerous dysrhythmia

    b. Unusual in healthy people

  5. Patient care management

    a. Monitor for cardiac irritability that may precipitate life-threatening dysrhythmias

    b. Treat or eliminate the underlying cause

O. Premature ventricular contraction (PVC)

  1. Definition: ectopic beat originating from a stimulus in the ventricles that occurs earlier than the normally expected beat and that is usually followed by a compensatory pause

  2. ECG characterisitics

    a. Rate: atrial and ventricular usually within normal limits but may be slow if many PVCs are present

    b. Rhythm: atrial and ventricular irregular because of the PVCs, but the underlying rhythm may be regular

    c. P wave: absent in the premature beat, unless retrograde conduction is present; then the P wave may follow the QRS complex

    d. PR interval: absent in the premature beat

    e. QRS complex: wider than 0.12 second and bizarre because the impulse arises from the ventricle in the premature beat

    f. ST segment: not considered because of abnormal depolarization of ventricles

    g. T wave: deflection is in the opposite direction of the widened QRS complex and is followed by a long, compensatory pause in the premature beat

  3. Possible causes

    a. Digitalis toxicity

    b. Hypokalemia

   c. Hypocalcemia
   d. Hypoxia
   e. Caffeine, tobacco, or alcohol ingestion
   f. Sympathomimetic drugs, such as epinephrine and isoproterenol
   g. Irritation of the myocardium by pacemaker electrodes
   h. Exercise above normal tolerance levels
 4. Clinical significance
   a. Decreased cardiac output because of a PVC
   b. In ischemic heart disease, PVCs are more likely to stimulate ventricular tachycardia, flutter, or fibrillation
   c. Dangerous forms include two or more in a row, bigeminy (every other beat is a PVC), multifocal (more than one irritable foci), more than six occurring in 1 minute, and R-on-T phenomenon
 5. Patient care management
   a. Do not treat if PVCs are rare and patient is otherwise healthy
   b. Administer oxygen if hypoxia is a cause
   c. Administer electrolyte replacement if imbalance is a cause
   d. Administer atropine if rhythm is bradycardic
   e. Administer antiarrhythmics, such as lidocaine, to decrease irritability

P. Ventricular tachycardia
 1. Definition: more than three PVCs occurring in succession at a rate of more than 100 beats/minute
 2. ECG characteristics
   a. Rate: atrial cannot be determined; ventricular is usually more rapid (100 to 250 beats/minute)
   b. Rhythm: atrial cannot be determined; ventricular is usually regular or slightly irregular
   c. P wave: usually not visible but may be retrograde
   d. PR interval: cannot be identified
   e. QRS complex: wide and bizarre; may resemble PVCs recorded before tachycardia began
   f. ST segment: difficult or impossible to determine
   g. T wave: deflection in the opposite direction of QRS complex
 3. Possible causes
   a. Myocardial ischemia or infarction
   b. Rheumatic heart disease
   c. Mitral valve prolapse
   d. CHF
   e. Cardiomyopathy
   f. Pulmonary embolism
   g. Electrolyte imbalance
   h. Drug toxicity from digitalis, procainamide, quinidine, or epinephrine

4. Clinical significance
   a. Life-threatening
   b. May deteriorate to ventricular fibrillation
5. Patient care management
   a. Do not plan to treat asymptomatic bursts of ventricular tachycardia that spontaneously convert
   b. Administer antiarrhythmics to decrease ventricular irritability
   c. If the patient is hemodynamically unstable, immediately defibrillate with 200 joules or watt-seconds
   d. Initiate basic cardiac life support (BCLS) and advanced cardiac life support (ACLS) protocols according to institutional policy
   e. Prepare the patient for overdrive pacing, which may be considered if bradycardia is a causative factor
   f. Prepare the patient for implantation of an automatic defibrillator, which may be considered if he does not respond to drug therapy

Q. Ventricular fibrillation
   1. Definition: rapid, disorganized depolarization of the ventricles, characterized by a lack of specific electrical impulse, conduction, and contraction
   2. ECG characteristics
      a. Rate: cannot be determined
      b. Rhythm: rapid and chaotic with no pattern or regularity
      c. P wave: not identifiable
      d. PR interval: not identifiable
      e. QRS complex: not identifiable
      f. ST segment: not identifiable
      g. T wave: not identifiable
   3. Possible causes
      a. MI
      b. Untreated ventricular tachycardia
      c. Electrolyte imbalance
      d. Electric shock
      e. Hypothermia
      f. R-on-T phenomenon
   4. Clinical significance
      a. Life-threatening
      b. Cardiac output stops and death follows quickly
   5. Patient care management
      a. Defibrillate immediately with 200 joules or watt-seconds
      b. Initiate BCLS and ACLS protocols according to institutional policy

R. Asystole (ventricular standstill)
1. Definition: total absence of ventricular electrical activity
2. ECG characteristics
   a. Rate: atrial usually indiscernible but could be present within normal limits; ventricular indiscernible
   b. Rhythm: atrial and ventricular usually indiscernible
   c. P wave: may be present
   d. PR interval: not measurable
   e. QRS complex: absent
   f. ST segment: absent
   g. T wave: absent
3. Possible causes
   a. Acute respiratory failure
   b. Severe metabolic deficit
   c. Extensive myocardial damage from ischemia, infarction, rupture, or aneurysm
4. Clinical significance
   a. Life-threatening
   b. Least responsive of lethal dysrhythmias
5. Patient care management
   a. Initiate BCLS and ACLS protocols according to institutional policy
   b. Defibrillate if unable to distinguish asystole from fine ventricular fibrillation
   c. Prepare the patient for insertion of a temporary pacemaker

Points to Remember

Digitalis toxicity should be considered as a possible cause for dysrhythmia in any patient taking the drug.

Dangerous forms of PVCs include two or more in a row, bigeminy, multifocal, more than six in 1 minute, and R-on-T phenomenon.

Immediate defibrillation is indicated for unstable ventricular tachycardia or ventricular fibrillation.

BCLS and ACLS protocols should be implemented according to institutional policies for all life-threatening dysrhythmias.

Glossary

Bigeminy—rhythm in which every other beat is a PVC

Cardioversion—timed or synchronized depolarization of the myocardial cells by an externally applied electrical charge

Defibrillation—untimed depolarization of the myocardial cells by an externally applied electrical charge

Dysrhythmia—abnormal cardiac rhythm; also called arrhythmia

R-on-T phenomenon—premature depolarization (R wave) that occurs during the relative refractory period of repolarization (T wave) of the preceding cycle; can trigger ventricular tachycardia or fibrillation

Cardiovascular Disorders

Learning Objectives

After studying this section, the reader should be able to:

● Describe the general principles of cardiovascular function.

● Identify the possible causes for each type of alteration in cardiovascular function.

● Discuss common assessment and diagnostic test findings for the patient with a specific alteration in cardiovascular function.

● Describe care management for the patient with a specific alteration in cardiovascular function.

XII. Cardiovascular Disorders

A. Basic concepts

1. The heart's function is to pump blood to the tissues, supplying oxygen and removing carbon dioxide and other metabolic waste products
2. Cardiovascular disease is the leading cause of death in the United States
3. Risk factors associated with increased risk of developing cardiovascular disease are classified as nonmodifiable, modifiable, or contributing
4. *Nonmodifiable* risk factors include:
   a. Age: cardiovascular disease increases with age
   b. Sex: men have a greater risk of developing cardiovascular disease than women do
   c. Race: nonwhites have a greater risk of developing cardiovascular disease than whites do
5. *Modifiable* risk factors include:
   a. Cigarette smoking
   b. Hypertension
   c. Increased serum cholesterol levels
   d. Diabetes
6. *Contributing* risk factors include:
   a. Obesity
   b. Physical inactivity
   c. Type A personality
   d. Stress
7. *Potential* nursing diagnoses for the patient with cardiovascular disorders include:
   a. Altered comfort: pain
   b. Altered cardiac output: decreased
   c. Activity intolerance
   d. Anxiety

B. Anatomy and physiology

1. Blood supply to the heart is provided by the coronary arteries; much variation exists in the pattern of coronary artery and collateral branching, including:
   a. Right coronary artery
   b. Left main coronary artery with major branches of the left anterior descending and circumflex arteries
   c. Collateral arteries that connect two branches of a single coronary artery or branches of the right with branches of the left; normally present but greatly enlarged with hypoxia or chronic anemia
2. The cardiac cycle consists of diastole and systole
   a. *Diastole,* the filling phase, occurs as the ventricle receives blood from the atria to provide stroke volume; the coronary arteries are perfused during this phase

      b. *Systole,* the ejection phase, occurs when ventricular pressure exceeds aortic pressure; 90% of myocardial oxygen consumption (MVO_2) occurs during isometric contraction

  3. Myocardial oxygen supply is determined by:
      a. Coronary artery anatomy
      b. Diastolic pressure
      c. Diastolic time
      d. Oxygen extraction based on hemoglobin and partial pressure of oxygen in arterial blood

  4. MVO_2, which must be in balance with blood supply to the heart, is determined by cardiac output

  5. Cardiac output (CO) measures cardiac performance and is calculated by multiplying the heart rate (HR) times the stroke volume (SV):

$$CO = HR \times SV$$

  6. Stroke volume consists of preload, afterload, and contractility
      a. *Preload* is the ventricular filling pressure at the end of diastole; clinical indicators are central venous pressure (CVP) on the right side of the heart and pulmonary artery wedge pressure (PAWP) on the left; preload is related to Starling's law
      b. *Afterload* is the amount of pressure the left ventricle must overcome during systole to open the semilunar valves and eject blood; clinical indicators are pulmonary vascular resistance (PVR) on the right side of the heart and systemic vascular resistance (SVR) on the left
      c. *Contractility* relates to changes in the force of contraction independent of changes in myocardial fiber length or preload; it has no clinical indicators

  7. The heart uses compensatory mechanisms to increase cardiac output; these include:
      a. Increasing the heart rate
      b. Thickening the ventricular wall
      c. Increasing the ventricular chamber size

  8. As compensatory mechanisms fail to maintain cardiac output, decompensation occurs

  9. The normal aging heart can provide a normal cardiac output of 4 to 6 liters/ minute under normal conditions but may have limited compensatory ability to provide increased cardiac output demanded by physically or emotionally stressful situations

C. Angina pectoris
  1. General information
      a. Angina pectoris causes chest pain or discomfort from insufficient myocardial oxygen supply
      b. Angina may be classified as stable, unstable, or variant
      c. *Stable angina* is characterized by a consistent pattern of cause, intensity, and duration; the pain is relieved with rest or nitroglycerin

    d. *Unstable angina* is characterized by a change in the quality, duration, severity, or frequency of pain or by a change in the activity level that triggers pain

    e. *Prinzmetal's* (or *variant*) *angina* is an atypical pain caused by coronary artery vasospasm and often unrelated to activity or other stress

2. Causes

    a. Coronary thrombosis over high-grade lesion

    b. Coronary artery vasospasm

    c. Increased oxygen demands

    d. Decreased coronary artery perfusion pressure

    e. Decreased diastolic filling time

    f. Anemia

3. Assessment findings

    a. Pain or discomfort precipitated by physical exercise, stress, cold, heavy meals, or smoking

    b. Pain relief within 2 to 5 minutes from rest, nitroglycerin, or both

    c. Retrosternal chest pain that may radiate to the jaw, the shoulders, or down one or both arms

    d. Descriptions of tightness, squeezing, burning, or smothering rather than pain

    e. Expression of fear of impending doom

    f. Elevated blood pressure as a response to pain

    g. Decreased blood pressure if chest pain is caused by ischemia, which causes decreased cardiac output

4. Diagnostic test findings

    a. ECG: depressed ST segment, with or without T-wave inversion; elevated ST segment in Prinzmetal's angina during an episode of chest pain; absence of an ECG abnormality does not rule out disease

    b. Stress testing: CAD

    c. Cardiac catheterization: atherosclerotic changes in coronary arteries

    d. Complete blood count (CBC): anemia as the cause of chest pain

5. Patient care management goal: to relieve acute pain and reduce the cardiac work load

    a. Administer oxygen to relieve ischemia at a flow rate based on institutional policy and the patient's condition

    b. Assess and document continuous ECG rhythm, vital signs, mental status, and heart and lung sounds

    c. Assess and document pain characteristics: location, duration, intensity (have patient grade pain on a scale from 1 to 10), precipitating factors, relief measures, and any symptoms that indicate changes in these parameters

    d. Assess vital signs with complaints of chest pain, and compare to baseline

    e. Begin I.V. nitroglycerin titrated until acute pain is relieved; check blood pressure every 15 minutes or according to institutional policy; maintain systolic blood pressure greater than 90 mm Hg or according to institutional protocol; document the patient's response to therapy

    f. Administer I.V. morphine in small doses to relieve pain and decrease preload

    g. Give sublingual, oral, or topical nitroglycerin prophylactically for chronic pain

    h. Consider calcium channel blockers with Prinzmetal's angina to block the influx of calcium into the cell; calcium channel blockers produce vasodilation of coronary and peripheral arteries

    i. Use beta-adrenergic blockers to decrease myocardial oxygen demand by decreasing contractility, heart rate, and blood pressure

    j. Notify the doctor and obtain a 12-lead ECG at the onset of recurring chest pain

    k. Maintain activity restrictions based on the patient's activity tolerance, to reduce myocardial oxygen demands

    l. Begin the patient on a low-cholesterol, low-sodium diet to alleviate the modifiable risk factors

    m. Consider percutaneous transluminal coronary angioplasty (PTCA) to improve blood flow through the stenotic coronary arteries

    n. Remember that a coronary artery bypass graft (CABG) may be indicated when medical treatment has been unsuccessful, based on the patient's symptoms and the cardiac catheterization report

    o. Provide patient education, and ensure that the patient can recognize signs and symptoms necessitating medical attention (unrelieved chest pain after taking three nitroglycerin tablets sublingually 5 minutes apart)

    p. Work with the patient and family to identify the patient's risk factors and necessary life-style modifications

    q. Refer the family to appropriate sources for cardiopulmonary resuscitation (CPR) training

    r. Ensure that the family can activate the emergency medical system if any problems occur at home

C. Acute myocardial infarction

    1. General information

        a. Myocardial infarction (MI) causes the death of myocardial tissue from inadequate blood supply to the myocardium

        b. MIs are classified according to the layer of myocardial tissue involved or to the location of damage to the left ventricle

        c. A *subendocardial* or *nontransmural MI* is limited to the inner half of the ventricular muscle; a *transmural MI* involves the entire thickness of the myocardium

        d. An *anterior MI* usually involves occlusion of the left anterior descending coronary artery

        e. An *inferior* or *diaphragmatic MI* usually involves occlusion of the right coronary artery

    f. A *posterior MI* involves occlusion of the right coronary artery or circumflex branch of the left coronary artery and usually also involves the lateral or inferior wall of the left ventricle

    g. A *lateral MI* is relatively rare, with damage confined to the lateral wall, although it may occur in combination with an anterior MI

    h. Right ventricular infarction occurs when occlusion of the right coronary artery damages the right ventricle; it occurs most often with an inferior MI

    i. An anterior or lateral MI produces significantly higher mortality, more damage to the myocardium, more conduction disturbances, and increased occurrences of congestive heart failure and cardiogenic shock than does an inferior or posterior MI

2. Causes

    a. Occlusion of coronary artery blood flow from coronary thrombus over a high-grade lesion

    b. Coronary artery vasospasm

    c. Increased oxygen demands

    d. Decreased coronary artery perfusion pressure

3. Assessment findings

    a. Substernal crushing chest pain that may radiate to jaw, shoulders, back, or down one or both arms or may be asymptomatic

    b. Pain unrelieved by rest, position, or nitroglycerin and lasting longer than 30 minutes

    c. Dyspnea

    d. Hypoxia

    e. Diaphoresis

    f. Nausea or vomiting

    g. Anxiety

    h. Decreased blood pressure

    i. Increased temperature

4. Diagnostic test findings

    a. Serum creatine phosphokinase (CPK): CPK-MB isoenzyme elevation greater than established institutional criterion that begins 4 to 8 hours after infarction, peaks at 24 hours, and lasts for 72 hours after infarction

    b. Serum lactate dehydrogenase (LDH): LDH_1 greater than LDH_2; this isoenzyme pattern of elevation develops 12 to 24 hours after infarction, peaks at 36 to 72 hours, and returns to normal within 10 days of the infarction

    c. ECG: changes in leads over area of infarct: ST segment elevation (indicating injury to myocardial tissue), ST segment depression (in leads that view the opposite wall), T wave flattening and inversion (indicating ischemia of the myocardial tissue), and Q wave abnormalities (representing tissue death), which are clinically significant if the Q wave is greater than one-third of the total QRS height or more than 0.04 second wide

     d. Chest X-ray: cardiac enlargement and signs of left ventricular failure (pulmonary congestion); may also be normal

     e. Echocardiogram: abnormalities of left ventricular wall motion and valve competency

     f. Hemodynamic monitoring: increased pulmonary artery pressure (PAP), increased PAWP, decreased cardiac output, and increased SVR, depending on extent of the MI

6. Patient care management goal: to relieve acute pain, reduce the cardiac work load, prevent and treat dysrhythmias, and manage fluid imbalances and limit infarct size by reperfusion

     a. Administer oxygen to relieve ischemia at a flow rate based on institutional policy and the patient's condition

     b. Assess and document characteristics of pain: location, duration, intensity (have patient grade pain on a scale from 1 to 10), precipitating factors, relief measures, and associated symptoms

     c. Assess and document continuous ECG rhythm, vital signs, mental status, heart and lung sounds, urine output, and any signs or symptoms indicating changes in these parameters

     d. Assess vital signs with complaints of chest pain, and compare to baseline

     e. Begin I.V. nitroglycerin titrated until acute pain is relieved; check blood pressure every 15 minutes or according to institutional policy; and maintain systolic blood pressure greater than 90 mm Hg or according to institutional protocol; document the patient's response to therapy

     f. Administer I.V. morphine in small doses to relieve pain and to decrease preload and myocardial oxygen consumption

     g. Consider antiarrhythmic I.V. drug therapy prophylactically or as ordered, based on institutional policy; lidocaine is the drug of choice based on the American Heart Association's ACLS protocol

     h. Administer thrombolytic therapy with tissue plasminogen activator or streptokinase within the first few hours to lyse the clot after any chest pain suggesting an infarction

     i. Keep in mind that the doctor may order anticoagulants to prevent clot formation

     j. If a pulmonary artery catheter is in place, assess and document PAP, PAWP, cardiac output, and SVR, as ordered

     k. Run a 12-lead ECG when pain occurs and then daily for 3 days to evaluate any evolutionary changes associated with MI

     l. Monitor serum potassium levels, and report levels outside normal limits; potassium levels should be kept higher than 4.0 mEq/liter to reduce the risk of dysrhythmias

     m. Enforce activity restrictions to decrease oxygen requirements

     n. Maintain accurate intake and output records and daily weights to assess fluid status

     o. Begin the patient on a low-cholesterol, low-sodium diet to alter modifiable risk factors

p. Consider PTCA to improve blood flow through the stenotic coronary arteries
q. Remember that a CABG may be indicated when medical treatment has been unsuccessful, based on the patient's symptoms and the cardiac catheterization report
r. Provide patient education, and ensure that the patient can recognize signs and symptoms necessitating medical attention (unrelieved chest pain after taking three nitroglycerin tablets sublingually 5 minutes apart) and understands guidelines for resuming sexual activity after discharge
s. Work with the patient and family to identify the patient's risk factors and necessary life-style modifications (smoking cessation, stress management, diet modification)
t. Refer the family to appropriate sources for CPR training
u. Ensure that the family can activate the emergency medical system if problems occur at home

E. Congestive heart failure
1. General information
   a. Congestive heart failure (CHF) results from the heart's inability to maintain sufficient output to meet the body's metabolic demands
   b. CHF is classified as left ventricular (LV) and right ventricular (RV) failure
   c. *LV failure* occurs when the left ventricle cannot pump blood efficiently from the lungs to the systemic circulation
   d. Pressure increases in the lungs from the accumulation of blood; as this pressure exceeds the pulmonary capillary oncotic pressure, fluid leaks into the pulmonary interstitial space, causing pulmonary edema
   e. LV failure commonly occurs suddenly, making the compensatory mechanisms ineffective
   f. *RV failure* occurs when the right ventricle cannot pump blood efficiently from venous return into the pulmonary system
   g. As the pressure backs up in the systemic circulation, body organs become congested with venous blood
2. Causes: LV failure
   a. CAD
   b. Hypertension
   c. Cigarette smoking
   d. Obesity
   e. Increased stress
   f. Sedentary life-style
   g. Diabetes
3. Causes: RV failure
   a. Mitral valve stenosis
   b. Acute RV infarctions
   c. Pulmonary embolus

  d. COPD
  e. LV failure
4. Assessment findings: LV failure
  a. Moist cough with frothy sputum
  b. Dyspnea
  c. Crackles
  d. S_3 or S_4 heart sounds
  e. Anxiety
  f. Diaphoresis
  g. Decreased blood pressure
  h. Tachycardia
  i. Dysrhythmias
  j. Pulsus alternans
5. Assessment findings: RV failure
  a. Fluid retention
  b. Jugular vein distention
  c. Peripheral edema
  d. Decreased urine output
  e. Hepatojugular reflux
  f. Bounding pulses
  g. Ascites
6. Diagnostic test findings
  a. Chest X-ray: pulmonary congestion or cardiomegaly
  b. Arterial blood gas analysis: hypoxemia or respiratory alkalosis
  c. ECG: left and right ventricular hypertrophy or dysrhythmias
  d. Serum electrolyte studies: hyponatremia (dilutional) or hypokalemia
  e. CBC: decreased hemoglobin and hematocrit (dilutional or anemic)
  f. Hemodynamic monitoring: LV failure—increased PAP, PAWP, CVP, or RAP; decreased cardiac output. RV failure—increased PAP, CVP, or RAP; normal PAWP
7. Patient care management goal: to treat the underlying or precipitating factors and to reduce cardiac work load
  a. Provide oxygen to relieve ischemia at a flow rate based on institutional policy and the patient's condition
  b. Assess and document continuous ECG rhythm, vital signs, mental status, heart and lung sounds, urine output, and any signs or symptoms indicating changes in these parameters
  c. Maintain activity restrictions based on the patient's activity tolerance, to reduce myocardial oxygen demands
  d. Administer I.V. morphine in small doses to decrease venous return, preload, myocardial oxygen consumption, and pain
  e. Begin diuretics to decrease preload and blood volume
  f. Start digitalis to increase contractility and decrease heart rate
  g. Consider vasopressors to increase contractility and support blood pressure
  h. Use nitrates to decrease preload and pulmonary and cardiac congestion

      i. Use afterload-reducing agents to decrease SVR and to aid ventricular ejection

      j. If a pulmonary artery catheter is in place, assess and document PAP, PAWP, cardiac output, and SVR, as ordered

      k. Provide patient education, and ensure that the patient can recognize signs and symptoms necessitating medical attention (increased shortness of breath, weight gain, decreased activity tolerance, or change in pulse rate or rhythm) and that he understands dietary restrictions

      l. Refer the family to appropriate sources for CPR training

      m. Ensure that the family can activate the emergency medical system if any problems occur at home

F. Cardiomyopathy

  1. General information

      a. Cardiomyopathy is a subacute or chronic disorder involving an abnormality of the ventricular muscle that causes heart failure

      b. Classification is made by physiologic, pathologic, and clinical signs; cardiomyopathy is classified as dilated, hypertrophic, or restrictive

      c. *Dilated cardiomyopathy* demonstrates enlarged ventricular cavity, little or no hypertrophy of muscle wall, and decreased systolic ejection fraction

      d. *Hypertrophic cardiomyopathy* produces an abnormally stiff left ventricle that limits ventricular filling; thickening of the septum impairs blood outflow from the ventricle and is called idiopathic hypertrophic subaortic stenosis

      e. *Restrictive cardiomyopathy* leads to impaired ventricular stretch and diastolic filling

      f. Regardless of the category, the course of cardiomyopathy is progressive, leading to impaired left ventricular ejection, blood stasis in the ventricle and eventually the atrium, increased preload and afterload, and CHF

      g. Cardiomyopathy may also be classified according to etiology as primary or secondary

      h. *Primary cardiomyopathy* results from an unknown cause

      i. *Secondary cardiomyopathy* results from a systemic disorder

      j. When heart failure from cardiomyopathy progresses to a point beyond medical responsiveness, the only hope for the patient's survival is a heart transplant

  2. Causes

      a. Idiopathic origin

      b. Excessive alcohol intake

      c. Infections

      d. Hypertension

      e. Metabolic diseases

      f. Toxic responses

      g. Immune diseases

      h. Neoplastic heart disease

3. Assessment findings
   a. Dyspnea on exertion
   b. Hypotension
   c. Ischemic chest pain
   d. S_3 or S_4 heart sound
   e. Crackles
   f. Murmurs
   g. Paroxysmal nocturnal dyspnea
   h. Easy fatigability
   i. Cough
4. Diagnostic test findings: diagnosis is commonly made by ruling out other diseases
   a. Chest X-ray: pulmonary congestion or cardiomegaly
   b. ECG: atrial fibrillation, tachycardia, ventricular ectopy, or left axis deviation
   c. Echocardiogram: abnormalities of left ventricular wall motion, dilation of cardiac chambers, and valve competency
   d. Cardiac catheterization: rules out coronary disease as causative factor
5. Patient care management goal: to reestablish and maintain hemodynamic stability
   a. Administer oxygen to relieve ischemia at a flow rate based on institutional policy and the patient's condition
   b. Enforce activity restrictions to reduce myocardial oxygen demands
   c. Use vasodilators to decrease preload and afterload and to improve cardiac output
   d. Use diuretics to reduce preload and pulmonary congestion
   e. Consider inotropic agents to increase myocardial contractility
   f. Begin calcium channel blockers to decrease cardiac work load through vasodilation
   g. Consider beta blockers for hypertrophic cardiomyopathy, to reduce outflow obstruction during exercise
   h. Consider anticoagulants to prevent clot formation associated with atrial fibrillation
   i. If a pulmonary artery catheter is in place, assess and document PAP, PAWP, cardiac output, and SVR, as ordered
   j. Provide patient education, and ensure that the patient can recognize signs and symptoms necessitating medical attention (increased shortness of breath, weight gain, decreased activity tolerance, or change in pulse rate or rhythm) and understands that the disease is chronic and requires ongoing management and treatment
   k. Work with the patient to devise a plan for risk factor modification (such as alcohol abstinence or dietary restrictions)

G. Cardiac tamponade
1. General information
   a. Cardiac tamponade is a sudden accumulation of blood or fluid within the pericardial space, causing heart compression and interfering with cardiac filling and ejection
   b. The pericardial sac normally contains 10 to 30 ml of fluid that protects the myocardium; it has limited stretching ability
   c. Clinical manifestations depend on the rate of fluid accumulation
   d. A sudden addition of 50 to 100 ml of fluid can cause a rise in intrapericardial pressure
   e. As intrapericardial pressure exceeds CVP, the heart chambers and the coronary arteries are compressed
   f. When cardiac filling and ejection are impaired, cardiac output is decreased and tissue perfusion is compromised
   g. Circulatory collapse can occur if acute cardiac tamponade is not corrected immediately
2. Causes
   a. Blunt or penetrating trauma to chest
   b. Complications from central line placement, cardiac catheterization, pacemaker insertion, or angiography
   c. MI
   d. Acute pericarditis
   e. Malignant metastases to the pericardium
3. Assessment findings: depend on the rate of fluid accumulation
   a. Hypotension
   b. Tachycardia
   c. Cold, clammy skin
   d. Dyspnea
   e. Precordial pain
   f. Muffled heart sounds
   g. Jugular vein distention
   h. Pulsus paradoxus
   i. Anxiety
4. Diagnostic test findings
   a. ECG: ST segment elevation or nonspecific ST and T wave changes
   b. Chest X-ray: normal or enlarged cardiac silhouette or widened mediastinum
   c. Echocardiogram: right-to-left shift of intraventricular septum with inspiration; echo-free space in front of right ventricular wall and behind left ventricular wall
5. Patient care management goal: to reestablish and maintain hemodynamic stability
   a. Anticipate performance of pericardiocentesis to drain pericardial space of excess fluid

   b. Assess and document continuous ECG rhythm, vital signs, mental status, heart and lung sounds, urine output, and any signs or symptoms indicating changes in these parameters
   c. Consider pericardiostomy, to drain pericardial space
   d. Initiate I.V. volume therapy with fluids and volume expanders through a large-bore peripheral I.V. line to increase diastolic filling pressure for improved cardiac output
   e. Administer oxygen to correct hypoxia at a flow rate based on institutional policy and the patient's condition
   f. Consider inotropic agents to increase contractility
   g. Begin resuscitative measures if necessary

H. Hypertensive crisis
   1. General information
      a. Hypertensive crisis is a severe, fixed elevation of the resting arterial pressure, which may produce vascular necrosis as diastolic pressure exceeds 140 mm Hg
      b. The speed of increase in recorded pressure may be more destructive than the actual blood pressure
      c. The mortality associated with hypertensive crisis that is untreated for 1 year is 75%
   2. Causes
      a. Inadequately treated or untreated essential hypertension
      b. Poor compliance with treatment plan
      c. Renal disease
   3. Assessment findings
      a. Diastolic blood pressure above 140 mm Hg
      b. Throbbing headache
      c. Renal impairment
      d. Vision loss
      e. Confusion
      f. Signs of heart failure (moist cough with frothy sputum, dyspnea, crackles, or S_3 or S_4 heart sounds)
   4. Diagnostic test findings
      a. Blood pressure measurements: severely elevated
      b. Funduscopic eye examination: retinal changes (hemorrhages, exudates, narrowed arterioles, and papilledema)
      c. ECG: left ventricular hypertrophy
      d. Chest X-ray: cardiomegaly and pulmonary congestion if cardiac failure is present
   5. Patient care management goal: to reduce blood pressure rapidly and to prevent further hypertensive episodes
      a. Administer I.V. nitroprusside (the drug of choice) to cause immediate vasodilation
      b. Monitor blood pressure every 5 minutes or according to institutional policy during titration of medications

c. Use direct arterial pressure monitoring or automatic blood pressure cuff monitoring to evaluate blood pressure accurately and continuously and to prevent hypotension with drug titration

d. Administer nitroprusside, mixing the drug only in dextrose 5% in water; keep the bag protected from light; assess for possible thiocyanate toxicity (nausea, tinnitus, or fatigue); draw serum thiocyanate levels every 72 hours

e. Assess and document continuous ECG rhythm, mental status, heart and lung sounds, urine output, and any signs or symptoms indicating changes in these parameters

f. Evaluate changes in visual acuity by assessing the patient's ability to recognize objects and people

g. Consider I.V. diazoxide instead of nitroprusside to vasodilate arterial smooth muscle

h. Administer I.V. labetalol hydrochloride instead of nitroprusside to block alpha and beta sympathetic response

i. Begin oral antihypertensive therapy after acute episode is controlled so the patient can be weaned off I.V. drugs

j. Maintain bed rest to minimize oxygen requirements

k. Be aware that a patient admitted to the emergency or intensive care areas may have antihypertensive therapy inadvertently interrupted, which may cause a rebound elevation of blood pressure

l. Provide patient education, and ensure that the patient understands the importance of continuing treatment even when feeling well, can take accurate blood pressure readings and keep daily records as directed, and recognizes the importance of complying with prescribed activity after blood pressure is controlled

m. Work with the patient to devise a plan for risk factor modification (smoking cessation, stress management, or diet)

Points to Remember

The main compensatory mechanisms the heart uses to maintain cardiac output are increasing heart rate, thickening of the ventricular wall, and increasing the chamber size of the ventricle.

Cardiovascular disease remains the leading cause of death in the United States.

The diagnosis of myocardial infarction is based on patient history, signs and symptoms, cardiac enzyme levels, and ECG changes.

Evaluation of the cardiovascular disease risk factors is an essential part of any cardiovascular assessment.

Glossary

Cardiac output—measurement of cardiac performance, calculated by multiplying the heart rate times the stroke volume

Cardiomegaly—hypertrophy of the heart

Pulsus alternans—pulse characterized by a regular alteration of strong and weak beats

Risk factors—characteristic findings associated with increased prevalence of a disease; modifiable risk factors for cardiovascular disease include cigarette smoking, hyperlipidemia, elevated blood pressure, elevated blood glucose levels, obesity, inactivity, and stress

S_3 or S_4 heart sounds—abnormal heart sounds occurring during diastole that result from resistance to ventricular filling

Starling's law—principle stating that the force of contraction depends on the length of the heart wall's muscle fibers. The more the muscles are stretched, the greater the force of contraction within physiologic limits

Respiratory Disorders

Learning Objectives

After studying this section, the reader should be able to:

- Describe the general principles of respiratory system function.

- Identify possible causes for each type of alteration in respiratory function.

- Discuss common assessment and diagnostic test findings for the patient with a specific respiratory disorder.

- Describe care management for the patient with a specific alteration in respiratory function.

XIII. Respiratory Disorders

A. Basic concepts

1. The primary function of the respiratory system is to provide oxygen for all metabolic processes and to remove carbon dioxide (CO_2)
2. Most patients in critical care units have some degree of respiratory dysfunction
   a. A critically ill patient may not have the reserve or the normal compensatory mechanism to prevent pulmonary complications
   b. A critically ill patient may not be able to cough
3. Risk factors commonly associated with respiratory disorders include:
   a. History of airway obstruction from aspiration, inflammation, laryngitis, chronic lung disease, pulmonary edema, or near-drowning
   b. Thoracic restriction from trauma, flail chest, ruptured diaphragm, surgery, obesity, ascites, or arthritis involving the spinal column
   c. History of neuromuscular deficits, such as central nervous system depression from drugs or trauma, coma, polio, multiple sclerosis, or Guillain-Barré syndrome
   d. History of parenchymal disease caused by trauma to the lung tissue from contusion, tumors, or adult respiratory distress syndrome (ARDS, or shock lung)
   e. Disturbance of pulmonary perfusion from emboli or pulmonary hypertension
4. The major management goal for a patient with a respiratory disorder is to maintain a patent airway
5. Potential nursing diagnoses for a patient with a respiratory disorder may include:
   a. Impaired gas exchange
   b. Ineffective airway clearance
   c. Activity intolerance
   d. Anxiety
   e. Potential for infection

B. Anatomy and physiology

1. Adequate gas exchange is essential for proper functioning of all body systems
   a. Normal stimulus for respiration is an increase in partial pressures of carbon dioxide in arterial blood ($PaCO_2$)
   b. In chronic lung disease, the stimulus for respiration when $PaCO_2$ is consistently elevated is a decrease in partial pressures of oxygen (PaO_2)
2. Respirations are regulated by mechanical and chemical factors and are influenced by lung distensibility (compliance) and by the size of airways and the resistance to the flow they impart

3. The secondary functions of the respiratory system are:
   a. Regulation of acid-base balance through the expiration or retention of CO_2
   b. Expression of emotion, such as sighing or laughing
   c. Regulation of water balance and temperature control through water evaporation during respirations

C. Respiratory acidosis
1. General information
   a. Respiratory acidosis is not a disease but an acid-base imbalance that results from any condition that interferes with pulmonary gas exchange and causes retention of CO_2 (hypoventilation)
   b. The excess CO_2 then combines with water to form carbonic acid, increasing the carbonic acid level in the blood
   c. Respiratory acidosis is classified as acute or chronic
   d. *Acute respiratory acidosis* is characterized by a sudden onset, with high $PaCO_2$ levels and a sharp decrease in serum pH that occur before the renal system begins to compensate (usually takes hours to days)
   e. *Chronic* (or *compensated*) *respiratory acidosis* is characterized by the body's adaptation to higher-than-normal CO_2 levels by the renal system, which allows retention of bicarbonate to balance the elevated level of carbon dioxide; produces a normal or near-normal pH
2. Causes
   a. Oversedation
   b. Neuromuscular disorders
   c. Trauma or surgery to the chest
   d. Obstructive lung disease
   e. Inappropriate mechanical ventilation
   f. Any condition contributing to hypoventilation
3. Assessment findings: early signs and symptoms are related to central nervous system depression
   a. Depressed rate and depth of respirations
   b. Tachypnea
   c. Headache
   d. Confusion
   e. Lethargy
   f. Dysrhythmias
   g. Dehydration
   h. Slow, deep respiration or coma
   i. Cyanosis
   j. Elevated intracranial pressure (chronic)
   k. Dilated conjunctival and facial blood vessels from hypercapnia (chronic)
   l. Edema from right ventricular failure (chronic)

4. Diagnostic test findings
    a. Chest X-ray: possible underlying pulmonary disease
    b. Arterial blood gas (ABG) measurements: uncompensated, pH less than 7.35, $PaCO_2$ greater than 45 mm Hg, HCO_3^- normal; compensated, pH normal, $PaCO_2$ greater than 45 mm Hg, HCO_3^- greater than 26 mEq/liter, PaO_2 less than 60 mm Hg (if hypoxia is a causative factor)

RESPIRATORY ACIDOSIS: A.B.G. FINDINGS

	pH	$PaCO_2$	HCO_3^-
Acute respiratory acidosis (uncompensated)	Below 7.35	Above 45	Normal
Chronic respiratory acidosis (compensated)	Normal	Above 45	Above 26

(*Note:* Your institution's laboratory values may differ slightly.)

    c. ECG: dysrhythmias present with acidosis, hypoxia, or electrolyte imbalances
5. Patient care management goal: to support respiration and restore acid-base balance
    a. Intubate and mechanically ventilate the patient if he cannot maintain breathing
    b. Administer oxygen therapy if hypoxia is present (use caution if hypoxia is a stimulus to breathe and the patient is not on mechanical ventilation)
    c. Suction as necessary to remove secretions
    d. Administer bronchodilators to dilate smooth muscles of large airways
    e. Administer antibiotics appropriate for causative organism, if infection is present
    f. Avoid use of narcotics and sedatives to prevent depression of respiratory center
    g. Avoid use of bicarbonate unless a base deficit exists
    h. Assess and document continuous ECG rhythm; vital signs; mental status; heart, lung, and bowel sounds; urine output; and any signs and symptoms indicating changes in these parameters
    i. Obtain ABG measurements and monitor for hypoxemia, hypercarbia, and acid-base imbalance
    j. Monitor laboratory results and report all abnormal values (serum potassium [K^+] may decrease as acidosis is reversed)
    k. Position the patient for comfort; elevate the head of the bed to facilitate gas exchange
    l. Have the patient turn, cough, and deep-breathe to aid gas exchange and perfusion

    m. Provide emotional support to decrease fear and anxiety
    n. Teach the patient to recognize the signs and symptoms of the disease requiring medical attention
    o. Teach the patient techniques for improving lung function, such as deep or pursed-lip breathing

D. Respiratory alkalosis
  1. General information
    a. Respiratory alkalosis is not a disease but an acid-base imbalance that results from any condition that interferes with pulmonary gas exchange and causes excessive loss of CO_2 (hyperventilation)
    b. Excessive loss of CO_2 causes a corresponding loss of carbonic acid in the blood
    c. Respiratory alkalosis is classified as acute or chronic
    d. *Acute respiratory alkalosis* is characterized by a sudden onset, with low $PaCO_2$ levels and a sharp increase in serum pH that occur before the renal system begins to compensate (usually takes hours to days)
    e. *Chronic* (or *compensated*) *respiratory alkalosis* is characterized by the body's adaptation to lower-than-normal CO_2 levels by the renal system, which allows excretion of bicarbonate to balance the decrease in CO_2; produces a normal or near-normal pH
  2. Causes
    a. Anxiety
    b. Hyperventilation
    c. Pulmonary emboli
    d. Pulmonary edema
    e. Fever
    f. Sepsis
    g. Salicylate poisoning or overdose
    h. Excessive mechanical ventilation
    i. Pregnancy
    j. Chronic hepatic insufficiency
  3. Assessment findings: early signs and symptoms are related to excitability of the peripheral and central nervous systems; chronic respiratory alkalosis is usually asymptomatic
    a. Increased rate and depth of respirations
    b. Dizziness
    c. Numbness or tingling in fingers and toes
    d. Sweating
    e. Muscle weakness
    f. Tetany
    g. Seizures
    h. Syncope
    i. Dysrhythmias

4. Diagnostic test findings
    a. Chest X-ray: possible underlying pulmonary disease
    b. ABG measurements: uncompensated, pH greater than 7.45, $PaCO_2$ less than 35 mm Hg, HCO_3^- normal; compensated, pH normal, $PaCO_2$ less than 35 mm Hg, HCO_3^- less than 22 mEq/liter, PaO_2 less than 60 mm Hg (if hypoxia is a causative factor)

RESPIRATORY ALKALOSIS: A.B.G. FINDINGS

	pH	Paco₂	HCO₃⁻
Acute respiratory alkalosis (uncompensated)	Above 7.45	Below 35	Normal
Chronic respiratory alkalosis (compensated)	Normal	Below 35	Below 22

(*Note:* Your institution's laboratory values may differ slightly.)

    c. ECG: dysrhythmias with alkalosis, hypoxia, or electrolyte imbalance
5. Patient care management goal: to support respiration and restore acid-base balance
    a. Use a rebreather mask or reservoir to increase the CO_2 level
    b. Administer oxygen therapy if hypoxia is present
    c. Administer sedatives or analgesics if anxiety or pain is a causative factor
    d. Consider changing the delivery mode of mechanical ventilation or parameter settings for tidal volume and rate
    e. Provide emotional support to decrease fear and anxiety
    f. Assess and document continuous ECG rhythm; vital signs; mental status; heart, lung, and bowel sounds; urine output; and any signs and symptoms indicating changes in these parameters
    g. Obtain ABG measurements and monitor for hypoxemia and acid-base imbalances
    h. Monitor laboratory results and report all abnormal values (serum K^+ may increase as alkalosis is reversed)
    i. Teach the patient relaxation techniques to decrease anxiety

E. Pneumonia
1. General information
    a. Pneumonia is a bacterial, viral, or fungal infection that causes inflammation of the lung tissue
    b. Pneumonia commonly impairs gas exchange
    c. Pneumonia is classified according to etiology (bacterial, viral, or fungal), location (bronchopneumonia, lobular, or lobar), or type (primary, secondary, or aspiration)

    d. Twelve to fifteen percent of all patients in critical care areas contract pneumonia

    e. Risk is increased in an elderly, immunocompromised, or chronically ill patient

    f. Onset of signs and symptoms is influenced by age, extent of disease, and causative organism

2. Causes
   a. Aspiration
   b. Administration of steroids
   c. Prolonged oxygen therapy
   d. Immobility

3. Assessment findings
   a. Productive or non-productive cough (may be suppressed in a critically ill patient)
   b. Mucoid, rusty, bloody, or purulent sputum
   c. Fever
   d. Chills
   e. Pleuritic pain
   f. Tachypnea
   g. Tachycardia
   h. Nasal flaring
   i. Use of accessory muscles for breathing
   j. Inspiratory crackles

4. Diagnostic test findings
   a. Chest X-ray: pleural effusion, consolidation, and inflammation
   b. Sputum analysis for culture and sensitivity: identification of causative organism for effective antibiotic
   c. White blood cell count: elevated in bacterial infection and normal or decreased in viral or mycoplasmic infection
   d. ABG measurements: hypoxemia and acid-base imbalances
   e. Blood culture: bacteria in the blood

5. Patient care management goal: to treat the infection and restore adequate ventilation for tissue perfusion
   a. Administer oxygen therapy if hypoxia is present
   b. Intubate and mechanically ventilate the patient if he cannot maintain breathing
   c. Suction as necessary to remove secretions
   d. Administer I.V. fluids for hydration and antibiotic therapy
   e. Administer antibiotics appropriate for the causative organism
   f. Administer antipyretics as necessary
   g. Administer analgesics for pleuritic pain
   h. Assess and document continuous ECG rhythm; vital signs; mental status; heart, lung, and bowel sounds; urine output; and any signs and symptoms indicating changes in these parameters
   i. Monitor sputum production for color, viscosity, and quantity
   j. Hydrate with I.V. and oral fluids but avoid overload

      k. Prevent transmission of infection by washing hands thoroughly and by wearing gloves when contact with blood or body fluids is likely

      l. Observe isolation procedures and precautions as defined by the Centers for Disease Control and institutional policy

     m. Teach the patient techniques for improving lung function, such as deep breathing, coughing, or spirometry exercises

     n. Help the patient identify the need for therapeutic assistance to stop smoking, if necessary

F. Status asthmaticus

1. General information
   a. Status asthmaticus is a severe, prolonged asthma attack that does not respond to traditional therapy of epinephrine and aminophylline
   b. Onset may be rapid but usually is gradual, occurring over several days
   c. Status asthmaticus is characterized by airway obstruction resulting from a spasm of the bronchial smooth muscle, mucosal edema, and the hypersecretion of mucus
   d. Obstructed airways interfere with gas exchange and increase airway resistance

2. Causes
   a. Failure to take prescribed asthma medications
   b. Exposure to allergens, such as smoke or dust
   c. Respiratory infections
   d. Stress

3. Assessment findings
   a. Extreme dyspnea with prolonged expiration
   b. Nasal flaring
   c. Use of accessory muscles
   d. Diminished breath sounds
   e. Prolonged wheezing on expiration; absence of wheezing indicates insufficient airflow and respiratory collapse
   f. Nonproductive cough (in acute phase)
   g. Tachypnea
   h. Tachycardia
   i. Chest tightness
   j. Fatigue
   k. Anxiety or fear

4. Diagnostic test findings
   a. Chest X-ray: hyperinflation
   b. ABG measurements: initially, severe hypoxemia, a normal pH, and a low $PaCO_2$ because of hyperventilation; followed by an elevation in $PaCO_2$ and a decrease in pH
   c. Pulmonary function tests: decreased forced vital capacity and forced expiratory volume

d. Complete blood count: increased eosinophils (indicate allergic response if the patient is not on steroids)

e. Sputum analysis for culture and sensitivity: identification of causative organism if infection is present

5. Patient care management goal: to restore adequate ventilation for tissue perfusion

a. Administer oxygen therapy to correct hypoxia

b. Intubate and mechanically ventilate the patient if he cannot maintain breathing

c. Suction as necessary to remove secretions

d. Administer I.V. fluids for hydration and medication therapy

e. Administer bronchodilators to dilate smooth muscles of large airways

f. Administer corticosteroids to decrease inflammatory response

g. Administer antibiotics appropriate for the causative organism, if infection is present

h. Administer sedatives or tranquilizers for agitation, if necessary, to encourage the patient's cooperation with therapy, such as mechanical ventilation

i. Assess and document continuous ECG rhythm; vital signs; mental status; heart, lung, and bowel sounds; urine output; and any signs and symptoms indicating changes in these parameters

j. Obtain ABG measurements and monitor for hypoxemia and acid-base imbalance

k. Monitor sputum production for color, viscosity, and quantity

l. Position the patient for comfort; elevate the head of the bed to facilitate respiration

m. Have the patient turn, cough, and deep breathe to aid gas exchange and perfusion

n. Provide emotional support to decrease fear and anxiety

o. Help the patient and family to identify allergens or irritants that may precipitate an attack

G. Pulmonary embolism

1. General information

a. Pulmonary embolism (PE) is a blockage of a pulmonary artery by foreign matter, such as a thrombus, fat, tumor, tissue, air, amniotic fluid, or particulate matter, such as a catheter fragment

b. Substances released from the blockage cause constriction of the bronchial passages decreasing lung volume and compliance

c. Hypoxemia arises from ventilation/perfusion (V/Q) mismatch

d. Alveolar collapse and atelectasis develop because the alveoli cannot produce enough surfactant to maintain alveolar integrity; these factors increase pulmonary artery pressure (PAP) and intrapulmonary shunting

e. PE is one of the most common acute respiratory disorders in hospitalized patients

      f. Nearly one-half of the PEs that cause death are undiagnosed

      g. Onset of signs and symptoms usually is sudden and requires prompt detection and intervention

2. Causes

      a. Stasis of the blood because of immobility

      b. Deep vein thrombosis

      c. Clotting abnormalities

      d. Atrial fibrillation

      e. Myocardial infarction

      f. Pelvic or abdominal surgery

      g. Pregnancy or estrogen therapy

      h. Trauma caused by long bone fractures (fat emboli)

3. Assessment findings

      a. Sharp, sudden pleuritic chest pain

      b. Dyspnea

      c. Tachypnea with splinting

      d. Restlessness and anxiety

      e. Cough with possible hemoptysis

      f. Tachycardia

      g. Petechiae on anterior chest, neck, and axilla if the source is a fat embolus

      h. Fever and diaphoresis

      i. S_3 or S_4 heart sounds

      j. Pleural friction rub

      k. Positive Homans' sign

4. Diagnostic test findings

      a. Chest X-ray: may be normal

      b. ABG measurements: hypoxemia and acid-base imbalances

      c. ECG: right axis deviation; tall, peaked T waves; S-T segment changes; and T-wave inversion in V_1-V_4 leads

      d. V/Q scans: ventilation/perfusion mismatch (interruption of blood flow to affected lung area)

      e. Pulmonary angiography (the definitive test but invasive): location and extent of embolus

      f. Hemodynamic monitoring: increased pulmonary vascular resistance evidenced by elevated PAP

5. Patient care management goal: to restore normal tissue perfusion and decrease the risk of further obstruction

      a. Administer oxygen therapy to correct hypoxia

      b. Prepare the patient for pulmonary artery catheter placement to monitor fluid levels and evaluate therapy

      c. Assess and document central venous pressure (CVP), PAP, pulmonary artery pressure (PAWP), cardiac output (CO), pulmonary vascular resistance (PVR), and systemic vascular resistance (SVR)

   d. Assess and document continuous ECG rhythm; vital signs; mental status; heart, lung, and bowel sounds; urinary output; and any signs and symptoms indicating changes in these parameters
   e. Administer I.V. heparin (treatment of choice if the source of the embolus is a clot) with initial bolus and maintenance by continuous drip or intermittent dosing for 7 to 10 days; administer oral agents concomitantly with heparin for 3 to 4 days before switching to oral agents alone
   f. Administer steroids to decrease local injury to tissue and to decrease pulmonary edema if the source is a fat embolus
   g. Monitor coagulation studies (partial thromboplastin time for heparin and prothrombin time for oral agents) to maintain levels at 1½ to 2 times normal values
   h. Obtain ABG measurements and monitor for hypoxemia and acid-base imbalances
   i. Position the patient for comfort; elevate the head of the bed to facilitate gas exchange; avoid bending at the knee
   j. Have the patient turn, cough, and deep breathe to aid gas exchange and perfusion
   k. Avoid I.M. injections to decrease risk of hematoma
   l. Provide a safe environment to prevent falls and injury to tissue
   m. Monitor the patient for signs and symptoms of bleeding secondary to anticoagulant therapy
   n. Apply antiembolism stockings; remove at night and put on again before the patient ambulates in the morning
   o. Prepare the patient for thrombolytic therapy with streptokinase or urokinase (used to speed lysis of clot, especially in hemodynamically compromised patients or those with large or multiple emboli)
   p. Prepare the patient for embolectomy, which may be required to remove massive embolus; mortality rate of procedure exceeds 50%
   q. Prepare the patient for surgical placement of a filter to prevent further movement of the thrombus (in selected patients)
   r. Teach the patient the importance of preventing venous stasis by avoiding prolonged standing or sitting (especially with crossed legs), or the use of oral contraceptives
   s. Teach the patient the importance of avoiding over-the-counter medications that may interfere with oral anticoagulant therapy

H. Adult respiratory distress syndrome
   1. General information
      a. Adult respiratory distress syndrome (ARDS) is noncardiogenic pulmonary edema caused by diffuse injury to the alveolar capillary membrane
      b. It is known by other names, such as shock lung, white lung, and DaNang lung
      c. ARDS mortality exceeds 50%

    d. ARDS is characterized by phases, beginning with a precipitating event or insult that is followed by a progressive decrease in pulmonary compliance, decreased surfactant production, interstitial edema, refractory hypoxia, and widespread areas of consolidation

2. Causes
   a. Trauma
   b. Shock
   c. Infection (especially gram-negative organisms)
   d. Air embolism, fat embolism, or thromboembolism
   e. Disseminated intravascular coagulopathy
   f. Aspiration
   g. Near drowning
   h. Oxygen toxicity
   i. Massive blood transfusions
   j. Cardiopulmonary bypass

3. Assessment findings
   a. Labored breathing (early)
   b. Restlessness (early)
   c. Dry cough (early)
   d. Clear breath sounds (early)
   e. Adventitious breath sounds (late)
   f. Cyanosis (late)
   g. Pallor (late)
   h. Agitation (late)
   i. Confusion (late)
   j. Accessory muscle retraction (late)
   k. Diaphoresis (late)

4. Diagnostic test findings
   a. Chest X-ray: normal in early phases; progressing to bilateral diffuse infiltrates, then to "white out," which is evidence of very little air in the lungs and characteristic of ARDS
   b. Pulmonary function tests: decreased compliance and lung volume and elevated peak inspiratory pressures
   c. ABG measurements: initially, respiratory alkalosis and hyperventilation; progresses to respiratory acidosis complicated by metabolic acidosis because of tissue hypoxia
   d. Sputum analysis: elevated albumin level from leakage of serum albumin into the alveolar space
   e. Hemodynamic monitoring: elevated PA systolic and diastolic pressures but a normal PAWP

5. Patient care management goal: to maintain adequate arterial oxygenation and pulmonary ventilation and to treat the underlying disease
   a. Intubate and mechanically ventilate the patient to relieve the work of breathing
   b. Administer oxygen therapy to correct hypoxia (may require a fraction of inspired oxygen [FIO_2] of 50% or greater)

    c. Use positive end-expiratory pressure (PEEP) to maintain adequate PaO_2 (may require 20 cm H_2O or greater)

    d. Suction as necessary to remove secretions

    e. Administer a paralyzing drug, such as pancuronium bromide (Pavulon), to further decrease the work of breathing and maximize use of mechanical ventilation

    f. Administer sedation with paralyzing drugs to decrease anxiety

    g. Administer corticosteroids to assist in stabilizing the cell membrane, which prevents escape of proteins and fluid into the interstitium

    h. Administer diuretic therapy to lower intravascular volume and to maintain a minimum PAWP to provide adequate CO

    i. Administer fluid therapy of colloids for patients who are hypoalbuminemic and crystalloids for all others

    j. Prepare the patient for pulmonary artery catheter placement to monitor fluid status and evaluate therapy

    k. Assess and document CVP, PAP, PAWP, CO, and SVR

    l. Assess and document continuous ECG rhythm; vital signs; mental status; heart, lung, and bowel sounds; urine output; and any signs and symptoms indicating changes in these parameters

    m. Administer nutritional support to meet the patient's metabolic needs and defend against infection

    n. Obtain ABG measurements and monitor for hypoxemia and acid-base imbalances

    o. Position the patient for comfort; elevate the head of the bed to facilitate respiration

    p. Have the patient turn, cough, and deep breathe to aid gas exchange and perfusion

    q. Provide emotional support to decrease fear and anxiety

    r. Encourage the patient to cooperate with efforts to support breathing

    s. Support the patient and family in their efforts to deal with the severity of the disease and the possibility of death

I. Exacerbation of chronic obstructive pulmonary disease

  1. General information

    a. Exacerbation of chronic obstructive pulmonary disease (COPD) presents as an acute episode when the obstruction increases to the point of severe respiratory distress

    b. If untreated, COPD leads to respiratory failure

    c. Classification of COPD includes asthma (see "Status asthmaticus," item F, in this section); emphysema, which occurs because of decrease in lung elasticity, causing air trapping; and chronic bronchitis, which results from inflammation and excessive mucus production

    d. COPD processes contribute to right ventricular failure and cor pulmonale

    e. Patients with COPD are usually critically ill before they become symptomatic

2. Causes
   a. Failure to take prescribed respiratory medications
   b. Infection
   c. Stress
   d. Cigarette smoking
   e. Trauma
   f. Respiratory irritants or allergens
3. Assessment findings: Emphysema
   a. Nonproductive cough
   b. Dyspnea
   c. Tachypnea
   d. Diminished lung sounds
   e. Use of accessory muscles for respiration
   f. Barrel chest
   g. Prolonged expiration
   h. Florid skin reflective of "pink puffer" syndrome
4. Assessment findings: Chronic bronchitis
   a. Productive cough with copious sputum
   b. Frequent infections
   c. Dyspnea
   d. Coarse wheezes and crackles
   e. Peripheral edema
   f. Cyanosis reflective of "blue bloater" syndrome
5. Diagnostic test findings
   a. Chest X-ray: hyperinflation with emphysema and congestion with bronchitis
   b. Pulmonary function tests: increased functional residual volume and decreased vital capacity and expired volumes
   c. ABG measurements: respiratory hypoxemia and respiratory acidosis
   d. Sputum analysis for culture and sensitivity: identification of causative organism for appropriate antibiotic
   e. ECG: right axis deviation and tachycardia
6. Patient care management goal: to maintain adequate arterial oxygenation and pulmonary ventilation and to treat underlying diseases
   a. Administer oxygen therapy to treat hypoxia (may require a low flow rate of 1 to 2 liters/minute to prevent depression of hypoxic drive as stimulus to breathe)
   b. Intubate and mechanically ventilate the patient if he cannot maintain breathing
   c. Suction as necessary to remove secretions
   d. Use PEEP to lower FIO_2 and facilitate weaning from the ventilator
   e. Prepare the patient for pulmonary artery catheter placement to monitor fluid status and evaluate therapy
   f. Assess and document CVP, PAP, PAWP, CO, PVR, and SVR

g. Assess and document continuous ECG rhythm; vital signs; mental status; heart, lung, and bowel sounds; urine output; and any signs and symptoms indicating changes in these parameters

h. Administer bronchodilators to dilate the smooth muscle of large airways

i. Administer antibiotics appropriate for the causative organism, if infection is present

j. Administer corticosteriods to decrease inflammation

k. Avoid the use of sedatives unless the patient is intubated and mechanically ventilated

l. Administer I.V. fluids for hydration and medication therapy

m. Provide nutritional support to meet the patient's metabolic needs and defend against infection

n. Obtain ABG measurements and monitor for hypoxemia and acid-base imbalances

o. Position the patient for comfort; elevate the head of the bed to facilitate respiration

p. Have the patient turn, cough, and deep breathe to aid gas exchange and perfusion

q. Provide emotional support to decrease fear and anxiety

r. Teach the patient who smokes the importance of stopping smoking

s. Help the patient to recognize the signs and symptoms of exacerbation of the disease and the need for medical follow-up

t. Teach the patient pursed-lip breathing to improve gas exchange

Points to Remember

Most patients in critical care or emergency areas have some degree of respiratory difficulty.

Oxygen therapy should be used with caution in patients who depend on hypoxia for the stimulus to breathe.

Narcotics depress the respiratory center.

Critically ill patients may not be able to cough.

Patients with chronic lung diseases may be critically ill before they become symptomatic.

Glossary

Compensation—effort by the renal system (requiring hours to days) to retain or excrete HCO_3^- to balance the effects of increased or decreased CO_2 levels, which present as respiratory acidosis or alkalosis

Hemoptysis—blood in sputum

Respiratory acidosis—acid-base imbalance occurring because of hypoventilation and retention of CO_2

Respiratory alkalosis—acid-base imbalance occurring because of hyperventilation and excessive loss of CO_2

Surfactant—substance formed in the lungs that reduces the surface tension to keep the alveoli open

Renal and Metabolic Disorders

Learning Objectives

After studying this section, the reader should be able to:

- Describe the general principles of renal and metabolic function.

- Identify possible causes for each type of alteration in renal or metabolic function.

- Discuss common assessment and diagnostic test findings for the patient with a specific alteration in renal or metabolic function.

- Describe care management for the patient with a specific alteration in renal or metabolic function.

XIV. Renal and Metabolic Disorders

A. Basic concepts

1. The kidneys' main function is to remove certain substances, including water, from the blood
2. Renal excretory function is necessary for the maintenance of life, but complete malfunction (unlike that of the cardiac and respiratory systems) may not cause death for several days
3. The renal system is adaptable to a wide variation in fluid load based on individual habits and patterns
4. The kidneys must be able to excrete substances that are digested and absorbed and not eliminated by other organs
5. Potential nursing diagnoses for a patient with renal or metabolic disorders include:
   a. Fluid volume excess (related to fluid overload)
   b. Fluid volume deficit (if caused by hypovolemia)
   c. Altered nutrition: less than body requirements
   d. Potential for infection

B. Anatomy and physiology

1. Key regulatory functions of the renal system include:
   a. Acid excretion
   b. Electrolyte excretion
   c. Water excretion
2. For the kidneys to excrete metabolic waste adequately, three conditions must occur:
   a. The kidneys must be adequately perfused
   b. The kidneys must function
   c. Urine must be released from the body
3. To excrete daily metabolic waste, normal kidneys must regulate renal blood flow at a constant level through autoregulatory mechanisms
4. Normally, 20% to 25% of resting cardiac output (CO) is distributed to the kidneys; as the mean arterial pressure falls below 60 mm Hg, autoregulation may be overcome and the kidneys may become hypoperfused
5. Diminished blood flow damages kidney tissue, impairing function
6. The kidneys regulate metabolic processes and maintain a steady balance between acids and bases that ensures optimal functioning of the cells
   a. Acids are continuously liberated as metabolic by-products, yet the pH is kept within a narrow range
   b. The narrow pH is maintained by the body's buffer systems, which prevent large changes in pH by chemically combining acids with other ions
7. Metabolic acid-base imbalances are produced when the body cannot maintain a steady balance
8. Metabolic imbalances produce respiratory compensation, which begins in minutes

C. Metabolic acidosis

1. General information
   a. Metabolic acidosis is an acid-base imbalance that occurs when acids increase and the normal acid-base ratio of 1:20 is altered
   b. Metabolic acidosis is not a disease but the result of increased acid production in the body or loss of bicarbonate
   c. Metabolic acidosis results from conditions that cause excessive fat metabolism in the absence of carbohydrates, anaerobic metabolism, underexcretion of metabolized acids, inability to conserve bases, and loss of sodium bicarbonate from the intestines
2. Causes
   a. Diabetic ketoacidosis
   b. Starvation
   c. Renal failure
   d. Poisoning
   e. Diarrhea
   f. Lactic acidosis
   g. Intestinal fistulas
   h. Administration of large amounts of normal saline or ammonium chloride
3. Assessment findings
   a. Tachypnea (Kussmaul's respirations)
   b. Headache
   c. Confusion
   d. Drowsiness
   e. Cold, clammy skin
4. Diagnostic test findings
   a. Arterial blood gas (ABG) measurements: uncompensated, pH less than 7.35, HCO_3^- less than 22 mEq/liter, $PaCO_2$ normal; compensated, pH normal, HCO_3^- less than 22 mEq/liter, $PaCO_2$ less than 35 mm Hg

METABOLIC ACIDOSIS: A.B.G. FINDINGS

	pH	HCO_3^-	$PaCO_2$
Acute metabolic acidosis (uncompensated)	Below 7.35	Below 22	Normal
Chronic metabolic acidosis (compensated)	Normal	Below 22	Below 35

(*Note:* Your institution's laboratory values may differ slightly.)

  b. Serum potassium: hyperkalemia

  c. Urinalysis: decreased urine pH (depends on etiology)

  d. ECG: dysrhythmias from acidosis or hyperkalemia

 5. Patient care management goal: to correct the metabolic defect

  a. Administer drugs to treat the underlying pathophysiologic processes, such as insulin for diabetes

  b. Consider sodium bicarbonate administration to restore normal HCO_3^- levels

  c. Remember that hemodialysis may be indicated for severe metabolic disturbances that risk death

  d. Monitor ABG measurements and serum electrolyte levels as needed for changes, and document the patient's response to therapy

  e. Employ continuous cardiac monitoring to detect cardiac rhythm disturbances

  f. Educate the patient and family about the risk factors and causative agents that should be modified, such as the misuse of medication or a delay in treating medical conditions

D. Metabolic alkalosis

 1. General information

  a. Metabolic alkalosis is an acid-base disturbance that occurs when bases increase and the normal acid-base ratio of 1:20 is altered

  b. Metabolic alkalosis is not a disease but the result of decreased acids in the body or an increase in HCO_3^-

  c. Metabolic alkalosis is produced from conditions that cause severe acid loss, decreased serum potassium and chloride, and excessive HCO_3^- intake

 2. Causes

  a. Vomiting

  b. Gastrointestinal suctioning

  c. Diuretic therapy

  d. Cushing's syndrome

  e. Excessive antacid ingestion

 3. Assessment findings

  a. Increased neuromuscular irritability

  b. Numbness or tingling of fingers and toes

  c. Tetany

  d. Seizures

  e. Dysrhythmias

  f. Hypoventilation

 4. Diagnostic test findings

  a. ABG measurements: uncompensated, pH greater than 7.45, HCO_3^- greater than 26 mEq/liter, $PaCO_2$ normal; compensated, pH normal, HCO_3^- greater than 26 mEq/liter, $PaCO_2$ greater than 45 mm Hg

METABOLIC ALKALOSIS: A.B.G. FINDINGS			
	pH	HCO$_3^-$	Paco$_2$
Acute metabolic alkalosis (uncompensated)	Above 7.45	Above 26	Normal
Chronic metabolic alkalosis (compensated)	Normal	Above 26	Above 45

(Note: Your institution's laboratory values may differ slightly.)

    b. Serum electrolytes: decreased potassium, calcium, and chloride
    c. Urine electrolytes: decreased chloride
    d. ECG: dysrhythmias from alkalosis or hypokalemia
  5. Patient care management goal: to correct the metabolic defect
    a. Administer drugs to treat underlying pathophysiologic processes, such as antiemetics for vomiting
    b. Infuse I.V. normal saline solution to replace fluid volume and chloride
    c. Administer potassium chloride to correct electrolyte imbalances
    d. Monitor ABG measurements and serum and urine electrolytes frequently for changes, and document the patient's response to therapy
    e. Employ continuous cardiac monitoring to detect cardiac rhythm disturbances
    f. Educate the patient and family about the risk factors and causative agents that should be modified, such as the misuse of medication or a delay in the treatment of medical conditions

E. Acute renal failure
  1. General information
    a. Acute renal failure (ARF) is a sudden deterioration in kidney function that results from the kidneys' inability to excrete water and metabolic wastes, leading to a progressive rise in creatinine and urea levels
    b. Renal failure is classified as prerenal, intrarenal, or postrenal, based on the underlying cause of failure
    c. *Prerenal* renal failure is caused by low perfusion to kidneys
    d. *Intrarenal* renal failure is caused by damage to the kidneys
    e. *Postrenal* renal failure is caused by an obstruction between the kidneys and the urinary meatus
    f. ARF can have a dramatic effect on fluid and electrolyte and acid-base balances
    g. The most common cause of ARF is acute tubular necrosis
    h. The key to ARF prevention is assessment of the patient at risk, including elderly, obese, and female patients, or those with underlying renal problems, chronic illness, or recent infections

      i. Certain drugs, primarily those excreted by the kidneys, require dosage modification in patients with ARF

2. Causes: prerenal
   a. Impaired cardiac function
   b. Hypovolemia
   c. Peripheral vasodilation
   d. Renal vascular obstruction
3. Causes: intrarenal
   a. Nephrotoxic drugs
   b. Infection
   c. Pigment release such as sepsis, transfusion reactions
   d. Rhabdomyolysis
   e. Obstetric complications such as eclampsia, septic abortion
   f. Other parenchymal disorders
   g. Prerenal conditions
4. Causes: postrenal
   a. Bladder obstruction
   b. Ureteral obstruction
   c. Urethral obstruction (prostatic hypertrophy)
5. Assessment findings
   a. Decreased urine output (less than 400 ml/day) for 1 to 2 weeks followed by diuresis sometimes exceeding 3 liters/day for 2 to 4 weeks, with a recovery period up to 1 year
   b. Weakness
   c. Increased blood pressure
   d. Dysrhythmias
   e. Kussmaul's respirations
   f. Peripheral edema
   g. Bleeding tendencies
   h. GI disturbances, such as anorexia, nausea, or vomiting
   i. Changes in level of consciousness, such as behavioral changes or confusion
   j. Muscle irritability
   k. Weight gain
   l. Pallor
6. Diagnostic test findings
   a. Serum chemistry: increased blood urea nitrogen (BUN), creatinine, potassium, phosphorus, and magnesium; decreased calcium, carbon dioxide, and sodium
   b. BUN:creatinine ratio: prerenal, greater than 20:1; intrarenal, 10:1; postrenal, 10:1
   c. Urine sodium: decreased (prerenal), increased (intrarenal), or normal (postrenal)
   d. Urine osmolality: increased (prerenal), decreased (intrarenal), or normal (postrenal)

    e. Urine specific gravity: increased (prerenal), fixed at 1.010 (intrarenal), or normal (postrenal)

    f. Urine sediment: normal (prerenal), casts and proteinuria (intrarenal), crystals (postrenal)

    g. Complete blood count: decreased hematocrit (HCT), hemoglobin, and red blood cells; increased prothrombin time and partial thromboplastin time

    h. ABG measurements: decreased pH and HCO_3^-

    i. Creatinine clearance test: less than 50 ml/minute

    j. Kidneys, ureter, and bladder (KUB) and flat plate of abdomen X-rays: rules out renal obstruction as a cause

    k. Intravenous pyelogram: rules out complete or partial urinary system obstruction

    l. Renal scan: decreased perfusion to the kidneys

7. Patient care management goal: to treat the underlying cause and correct metabolic disturbances

    a. Assess and document continuous ECG rhythm; vital signs; mental status; heart, lung, and bowel sounds; urine output; and any signs or symptoms indicating changes in these parameters

    b. Weigh the patient daily, at the same time and on the same scale

    c. Administer I.V. fluid therapy to correct fluid volume and electrolyte imbalances

    d. Administer low-dose dopamine (prerenal) to increase blood pressure and CO volume

    e. Assess for signs of fluid overload or hypovolemic shock

    f. Monitor serum chemistry for electrolyte imbalances

    g. Anticipate the need for I.V. calcium gluconate to counteract the toxic cardiac effects of hyperkalemia

    h. Administer calcium exchange resins, such as sodium polystyrene sulfonate orally or rectally, to lower serum potassium levels by removing potassium through the GI tract

    i. Administer diuretic therapy after the patient is adequately hydrated (prerenal)

    j. Determine the causative agent of intrarenal ARF, and discontinue any related antibiotics, analgesics, anesthetics, or pesticide exposure

    k. Institute dietary restrictions—including a diet low in protein, potassium, and sodium and high in carbohydrates—either orally, enterally, or parenterally

    l. Administer blood products to stabilize HCT and platelet count (intrarenal)

    m. Administer antibiotic therapy to treat the urinary infection, if present (postrenal)

    n. Prepare for possible dialysis if interventions are unsuccessful

    o. Document the patient's response to therapy

F. Electrolyte disturbances
1. General information
   a. Electrolyte disturbances occur when extracellular electrolyte concentrations fall outside normal levels
   b. Electrolytes serve many functions within the body, such as assisting with regulation of water and acid-base balance, affecting neuromuscular activity, and contributing to enzyme reactions
   c. As the electrolyte balance is disturbed, alterations in body functions occur
   d. The major electrolytes are sodium (Na^+), potassium (K^+), calcium (Ca^{++}), and magnesium (Mg^{++})
   e. Concentrations of intracellular and extracellular electrolytes differ: sodium is more abundant in extracellular fluid, whereas potassium is concentrated in intracellular fluid (ICF)
   f. Serum levels of electrolytes measure extracellular concentrations but may not always provide an accurate index of intracellular levels
   g. ECG changes are the most reliable indicators of potassium levels
2. Causes: see *Electrolyte disturbances*
3. Assessment findings
   a. An electrolyte imbalance reflects body function disturbances
   b. Signs and symptoms become more severe as electrolyte imbalances worsen
   c. See *Electrolyte disturbances* for specific information
4. Diagnostic test findings
   a. Serum levels of electrolytes: increased or decreased
   b. ABG measurements: acid-base disturbances
   c. ECG with hypokalemia: flattened T wave, depressed ST segment, prominent U wave
   d. ECG with hyperkalemia: widened QRS complex; tall, tented T wave; flattened P wave; depressed ST segment; prolonged PR interval; and asystole
   e. ECG with hypercalcemia: dysrhythmias and shortened QT interval
   f. ECG with hypocalcemia: prolonged QT interval
   g. ECG with hypermagnesemia: widened QRS complex, prolonged PR interval, elevated T wave
   h. ECG with hypomagnesemia: flattened T wave, slight widening of QRS complex, diminished voltage of P waves and QRS complex, prominent U wave
5. Patient care management goal: to correct the underlying cause of the electrolyte imbalance and return the electrolyte level to normal (see *Electrolyte disturbances* for specific management)
   a. Monitor intake and output to assess fluid status
   b. Monitor the ECG to observe for signs of continuing changes in cardiac rhythm or complexes

(Text continues on page 134.)

ELECTROLYTE DISTURBANCES

ELECTROLYTE DISTURBANCE	CAUSES	ASSESSMENT FINDINGS	PATIENT CARE MANAGEMENT
Hyponatremia (Na <135 mEq/ liter)	GI, skin, or renal losses; SIADH; CHF; oliguric renal failure	Abdominal and muscle cramps, anorexia, lethargy, confusion, seizures	Administer I.V. hypertonic saline solution (3% or 5% sodium chloride).
Hypernatremia (Na >145 mEq/ liter)	Osmotic diuresis, diabetes insipidus, saltwater near-drowning	Low-grade fever; flushed skin; weakness; thirst; dry, swollen tongue; disorientation	Administer water I.V. or by mouth to replace loss. Give diuretics and water I.V. or by mouth for sodium gain.
Hypokalemia (K <3 mEq/liter)	GI or renal losses, hyperaldosteronism, increased diaphoresis, diuretics	Fatigue, nausea, vomiting, muscle weakness, decreased bowel motility, anorexia	Administer potassium (K) I.V. or by mouth for replacement.
Hyperkalemia (K >5.5 mEq/liter)	Renal disease, potassium-sparing diuretics, tissue breakdown, acidosis, insulin deficiency	Muscle weakness, nausea, diarrhea	Give ion exchange resin to exchange sodium (Na) for K. Give I.V. glucose insulin and sodium bicarbonate (NaHCO$_3$) to drive K into cell temporarily. Give I.V. calcium (Ca) gluconate to block neuromuscular and cardiac effects.
Hypocalcemia (Ca <10.5 mg/dl)	Alkalosis, administration of banked citrated blood, impaired vitamin D absorption, hypoparathyroidism, decreased magnesium or phosphate	Tetany, seizures, positive Chvostek's and Trousseau's signs, tingling of fingers and mouth, memory impairment	Give Ca I.V. or by mouth for replacement. Give vitamin D by mouth to increase GI absorption of Ca. Give aluminum hydroxide by mouth to promote binding with phosphate.
Hypercalcemia (Ca >10.5 mEq/ liter)	Acidosis, renal failure, cancer or multiple myeloma, hyperparathyroidism, increased intestinal absorption	Muscle weakness, nausea, vomiting, anorexia, constipation, memory impairment	Administer normal saline I.V. to aid Ca excretion. Give phosphate I.V. to cause inverse drop in Ca. Encourage low-calcium diet. Administer steroids to alter vitamin D absorption. Promote weight bearing, if tolerated, to stimulate bone deposition. Give NaHCO$_3$ to treat acidosis.
Hypomagnesemia (Mg <1.5 mEq/ liter)	Alcoholism, GI loss, administration of banked citrated blood, osmotic diuresis	Tremors, difficulty swallowing, tetany, positive Chvostek's and Trousseau's signs, seizures, mood swings	Increase dietary intake of Ca. Administer magnesium sulfate I.V.
Hypermagnesemia (Mg >2.5 mEq/ liter)	Renal failure, excessive Mg administration, untreated diabetic ketoacidosis	Facial flushing, hypotension, respiratory depression, loss of deep tendon reflexes, coma	Administer Ca I.V. Prepare for dialysis. Institute mechanical ventilation if respiratory depression is significant.

E.C.G. CHANGES IN ELECTROLYTE IMBALANCES

A potassium, calcium, or magnesium imbalance—either an excess or a deficiency—will have a marked effect on a patient's cardiac conduction system, as shown on his ECG strip. Recognizing these ECG abnormalities may help prevent serious and possibly life-threatening problems.

Laboratory value:
Serum potassium > 5.5 mEq/liter

Tall, tented T wave—most prominent characteristic

Prolonged PR interval

Widened QRS complex   Flattened P wave   Depressed ST segment

HYPERKALEMIA

Laboratory value:
Serum calcium > 10.5 mg/dl

Shortened QT interval

HYPERCALCEMIA

Laboratory value:
Serum magnesium > 2.5 mEq/liter

Widened QRS complex

Elevated T wave

Prolonged PR interval

HYPERMAGNESEMIA

Laboratory value:
Serum potassium < 3 mEq/liter

Prominent U wave

Flattened T wave

Depressed ST segment

HYPOKALEMIA

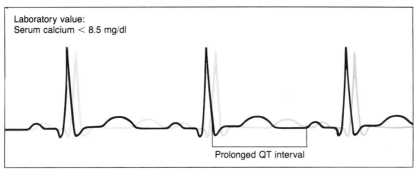

Laboratory value:
Serum calcium < 8.5 mg/dl

Prolonged QT interval

HYPOCALCEMIA

Laboratory value:
Serum magnesium < 1.5 mEq/liter

Diminished voltage of P waves

Diminished voltage and slightly widened QRS complex

Prominent U wave

Flattened T wave

HYPOMAGNESEMIA

c. Carefully reposition the patient with hypercalcemia because his bones may be brittle and fractures are probable

d. Assess the patient with hypercalcemia for signs and symptoms of kidney stone formation, such as hematuria, intermittent low back pain, and nausea or vomiting

e. Ensure that the patient with hypomagnesemia can swallow before administering oral medications or foods

f. Evaluate the patient with hypermagnesemia for changes in deep tendon reflexes

g. Be alert for the need of emergency intervention or mechanical ventilation if the patient develops respiratory depression from hypermagnesemia

h. Teach the patient to avoid over-the-counter medications that contribute to electrolyte imbalance

i. Document the patient's response to therapy

G. Fluid volume disturbances

1. General information

a. Fluid volume disturbances are alterations in the normal fluid balance within the body

b. Fluid disturbances can be caused by disease, illness-related changes in ingestion of fluid or food, or therapy

c. In the critically ill patient, the kidneys and other organs responsible for regulating fluid and electrolytes often fail, complicating the disturbance

d. When the compensatory mechanisms fail, the nurse plays a crucial role in calculating fluid gain or loss and administering fluid volume precisely

e. Failure to properly recognize and treat fluid disturbances in the critically ill patient can produce fatal complications

f. Fluid volume disturbances are of two major types: fluid volume excess and fluid volume deficit

g. *Fluid volume excess* reflects an increased accumulation of water and electrolytes in the extracellular fluid (ECF); it usually results from an increase in total sodium concentration, causing more water to be drawn into the ECF to re-establish the proper sodium-to-water ratio

h. *Fluid volume deficit* results from excessive loss of water and electrolytes from the ECF

i. Fluid volume deficit may be *isotonic* (sodium and water are lost in equal proportions), *hypertonic* (more water than sodium is lost or ECF concentration of sodium increases), or *hypotonic* (more sodium than water is lost or ECF concentration of water increases)

2. Causes: fluid volume excess

a. Fluid overload

b. Sodium overload

c. Diminished homeostatic mechanisms, such as those occurring in congestive heart failure, cirrhosis, or excessive corticosteroid therapy

3. Causes: fluid volume deficit
   a. Insufficient intake of water and electrolytes
   b. Excessive fluid loss through secretions or excretions
   c. Both conditions occurring simultaneously (most common)
   d. Third space shifting
4. Assessment findings: fluid volume excess
   a. Excessive weight gain (1 liter of fluid weighs about 2¼ lb)
   b. Elevated blood pressure
   c. Dyspnea
   d. Neck vein distention
   e. Elevated central venous pressure (CVP)
   f. Elevated pulmonary artery pressure (PAP)
   g. Dependent edema, may be pitting
   h. Bounding pulses
   i. Crackles
5. Assessment findings: fluid volume deficit
   a. Oliguria
   b. Dizziness
   c. Syncope
   d. Poor skin turgor
   e. Dry mucous membranes
   f. Hypotension
   g. Orthostatic blood pressure differences
   h. Decreased CVP, PAP, and CO
   i. Weakness
   j. Nausea and vomiting
6. Diagnostic test findings: fluid volume excess (related to hemodilution)
   a. BUN: decreased
   b. Complete blood count (CBC): decreased HCT levels
   c. Serum sodium: normal or decreased
   d. Serum and urine osmolality: decreased in patients with normal renal function
7. Diagnostic test findings: fluid volume deficit (related to hemoconcentration; may vary with type of fluid volume deficit)
   a. BUN:creatinine ratio: greater than normal ratio of 10:1
   b. CBC: increased HCT levels
   c. Serum sodium: increased (hypertonic), decreased (hypotonic), or normal (isotonic)
   d. Serum and urine osmolality: increased (hypertonic), decreased (hypotonic), or normal (isotonic)
   e. Urine specific gravity: elevated (may not occur for several hours)
8. Patient care management goal for fluid volume excess: to restore normal fluid volume to the ECF by treating the causative factors
   a. Administer diuretics to decrease fluid volume
   b. Maintain fluid restrictions to promote fluid balance
   c. Discontinue sodium-containing fluids to prevent further fluid retention

   d. Provide sodium-restricted diets to prevent further fluid retention
   e. Consider dialysis or continuous arterial-venous hemofiltration to quickly correct fluid overload
   f. Monitor intake and output hourly for changes
   g. Assess hemodynamic parameters, especially CVP and PAP, for changes
   h. Measure urine specific gravity as needed to evaluate the patient's fluid status and response to therapy
   i. Weigh the patient daily, at the same time and on the same scale, to evaluate fluid balance
   j. Monitor for signs of pulmonary edema, such as shortness of breath and dyspnea
   k. Evaluate for possible causative factors, such as heart failure, renal failure, burns, excessive glucocorticoid administration, or overzealous administration of I.V. fluids
9. Patient care management goal for fluid volume deficit: to restore normal fluid volume to the ECF and improve tissue perfusion
   a. Administer dextrose 5% in water (D_5W) for replacement; D_5W provides 170 calories/liter and shifts evenly between ICF and ECF
   b. Consider administering normal saline solution (0.9% sodium chloride) to expand ECF only, because it is an isotonic fluid that corrects mild sodium depletion
   c. Use albumin to expand the intravascular component of ECF and pull fluid into blood vessels from interstitial spaces
   d. Give blood to expand the intravascular component of ECF
   e. Consider vasopressors when the patient is adequately hydrated but his response to volume replacement is inadequate
   f. Monitor intake and output hourly to assess fluid balance accurately
   g. Assess hemodynamic parameters, especially CVP, PAP, and CO
   h. Measure urine specific gravity as needed to evaluate the patient's fluid status and response to therapy
   i. Weigh the patient daily, at the same time and on the same scale, to ensure accurate measurements
   j. Institute safety measures to prevent injury to the patient with altered sensorium
   k. Evaluate for possible causative factors, such as GI, skin, or renal losses; third space shifting; altered intake; or hemorrhage

Points to Remember

The renal system is responsible for regulating excretion of water, electrolytes, and acid substances.

A mean arterial pressure of 60 mm Hg is necessary for renal system autoregulation.

The most common cause of ARF is acute tubular necrosis.

Prevention of ARF is a primary goal in susceptible patients.

Metabolic acid-base imbalances are caused by an underlying disease that disrupts the normal acid-base ratio.

Major electrolyte imbalances can be life-threatening.

The most reliable indicators of ECF potassium imbalances are ECG changes.

Glossary

Autoregulation—ability of vessels to alter their diameter to balance blood flow with metabolic demands

Chvostek's sign—diagnostic sign of hypocalcemia; considered positive when a sharp tapping over the facial nerve just in front of the ear produces a twitching of the mouth, nose, and eye

Compensation—immediate effort by the respiratory system to retain or remove CO_2 to balance the effects of increased or decreased HCO_3^- levels, which present as metabolic acidosis or alkalosis

Nephrotoxic—substance destructive to the kidneys

Trousseau's sign—diagnostic sign of hypocalcemia; considered positive since ischemia produces carpopedal spasm when a blood pressure cuff is inflated above systolic blood pressure for 2 minutes

SECTION XV

Endocrine Disorders

Learning Objectives

After studying this section, the reader should be able to:

- Describe the general principles of endocrine function.

- Identify possible causes for each type of alteration in endocrine function.

- Discuss common assessment and diagnostic test findings for the patient with a specific endocrine disorder.

- Describe care management for the patient with a specific alteration in endocrine function.

XV. Endocrine Disorders

A. Basic concepts
1. The endocrine system regulates secretion of hormones that alter metabolic body functions, including:
   a. Chemical reactions
   b. Growth
   c. Transport of chemicals
2. Treatment involves restoring normal hormone production or secretion
3. Potential nursing diagnoses for a patient with endocrine system dysfunction may include:
   a. Altered tissue perfusion
   b. Fluid volume deficit or excess
   c. Altered nutrition
   d. Sensory-perceptual alteration

B. Anatomy and physiology
1. The endocrine system is closely related to the nervous system for regulation and control of specific hormones through its feedback systems involving the hypothalamus, pituitary gland, and target glands
2. Hormones act as chemical messengers; they:
   a. Are released directly into the bloodstream
   b. Act directly on the target organ
   c. Have a generalized effect on the entire body
3. Endocrine dysfunction involves either insufficient or excessive hormone production or secretion; causes include:
   a. Congenital or genetic defects
   b. Surgery
   c. Atrophy
   d. Neoplasms

C. Diabetic ketoacidosis
1. General information
   a. Diabetic ketoacidosis (DKA) is an emergency condition of hyperglycemia and ketonemia resulting from deficient insulin production or the cells' inability to use insulin
   b. DKA is the most common complication of diabetes mellitus
   c. In the absence of glucose, fat is broken down for energy; this results in ketonuria and ketonemia
   d. DKA can lead to severe dehydration and electrolyte depletion from osmotic diuresis, metabolic acidosis from hyperketonemia, and hyperosmolarity from hyperglycemia and dehydration
   e. Signs and symptoms develop quickly and require prompt attention
2. Causes
   a. History of uncontrolled diabetes mellitus Type I
   b. Infection
   c. Surgery

    d. Trauma

    e. Stress

    f. Pregnancy

    g. Decreased exercise

    h. Increased food intake without appropriate insulin adjustment

    i. Inadequate exogenous insulin administration

3. Assessment findings

    a. Dry, flushed skin

    b. Dehydration, evidenced by dry mucous membranes and poor skin turgor

    c. Fruity breath odor

    d. Kussmaul's respirations (rapid and deep)

    e. Polyphagia, polydipsia, or polyuria

    f. Fever

    g. Nausea, vomiting, or abdominal pain

    h. Altered level of consciousness (LOC) from irritability progressing to coma

4. Diagnostic test findings

    a. Serum glucose: 200 to 800 mg/dl

    b. Serum ketones: elevated

    c. Urine ketones: elevated

    d. Serum sodium: decreased

    e. Serum potassium: elevated initially, then decreased because of diuresis

    f. Arterial blood gas (ABG) measurements: pH reflects acidosis

    g. Hemoglobin (Hb) and hematocrit (HCT): elevated because of diuresis and dehydration

    h. Hemodynamic monitoring: pressures below the patient's normal baseline reflect dehydration

    i. ECG: dysrhythmias from potassium imbalance

5. Patient care management goal: to hydrate the patient and restore the acid-base balance

    a. Administer I.V. fluids (usually 0.9% or 0.45% saline solution) initially, given rapidly until serum glucose levels decrease to 200 to 300 mg/dl; then administer glucose solutions to prevent hypoglycemia

    b. Administer fluids through a large-bore peripheral I.V. to allow for rapid infusion

    c. Administer regular insulin first as a bolus, then as a continuous I.V. infusion to decrease serum glucose

    d. Administer I.V. potassium to replace serum potassium that returns to the intracellular fluid with the reversal of acidosis

    e. Prepare the patient for pulmonary artery catheter placement to monitor fluid status and evaluate therapy

    f. Assess and document central venous pressure (CVP), pulmonary artery pressure (PAP), pulmonary artery wedge pressure (PAWP), cardiac output (CO), and systemic vascular resistance (SVR)

g. Assess and document continuous ECG rhythm; vital signs; mental status; heart, lung, and bowel sounds; urine output; and any signs and symptoms indicating changes in these parameters

h. Insert a nasogastric (NG) tube to relieve gastric distention and prevent aspiration

i. Administer antibiotics to treat the underlying infection

j. Monitor and report any abnormalities in serum glucose and electrolyte levels

k. Obtain ABG measurements and monitor for hypoxemia and acid-base imbalance

l. Provide safety measures to prevent accidental injury from altered LOC

m. Position the patient for comfort; elevate the head of the bed to facilitate respiration and prevent aspiration

n. Teach the patient the causes of DKA

o. Teach the patient to recognize signs and symptoms of hyperglycemia requiring medical intervention

p. Instruct the patient in the proper technique for blood glucose testing to monitor diabetes, and have him demonstrate the technique

D. Hyperosmolar hyperglycemic nonketotic coma

1. General information

   a. Hyperosmolar hyperglycemic nonketotic coma (HHNC) is a life-threatening emergency caused by severe hyperglycemia but with an absence of ketone production

   b. Insulin is present in amounts adequate to prevent ketosis but not hyperglycemia

   c. Hyperglycemia is usually more pronounced in HHNC than in DKA

   d. The mortality from HHNC is about 60%

   e. Signs and symptoms may develop gradually, taking up to 2 weeks to become severe, and typically are nonspecific

2. Causes

   a. Undiagnosed diabetes mellitus Type II

   b. Stress

   c. Infection

   d. Acute pancreatitis

   e. Alcohol ingestion

   f. Trauma, such as head injury or burns

   g. Medical therapy, such as total parenteral nutrition, peritoneal dialysis, or hypothermia

   h. Medications, such as glucocorticoids, phenytoin, or diuretics

3. Assessment findings

   a. Severe dehydration, evidenced by dry mucous membranes and poor skin turgor

   b. Polydipsia and polyuria

   c. Altered LOC

   d. Hypotension

  e. Tachypnea with shallow respirations
  f. Profound weakness
4. Diagnostic test findings
  a. Serum glucose: elevated (may be greater than 800 mg/dl)
  b. Urinalysis: absence of ketonuria
  c. Serum sodium: elevated
  d. Serum potassium: normal or low
  e. Serum osmolality: elevated (greater than 350 mOsm/liter)
  f. ABG measurements: pH may be normal or mildly acidotic
  g. Hb and HCT: elevated because of dehydration
  h. Hemodynamic monitoring: pressures below the patient's normal baseline
     reflect dehydration
  i. ECG: dysrhythmias from potassium imbalance
5. Patient care management goal: to hydrate the patient and restore acid-base
   balance
  a. Administer I.V. fluids (usually 0.9% or 0.45% saline solution) initially,
     given rapidly until serum glucose levels decrease to 200 to 300 mg/dl;
     then administer glucose solutions to prevent hypoglycemia
  b. Administer fluids through a large-bore peripheral I.V. to allow for rapid
     infusion
  c. Administer regular insulin first as a bolus, then as a continuous I.V.
     infusion to decrease serum glucose
  d. Administer I.V. potassium to replace serum potassium that returns to the
     intracellular fluid with the reversal of acidosis
  e. Prepare the patient for pulmonary artery catheter placement to monitor
     fluid status and evaluate therapy
  f. Assess and document CVP, PAP, PAWP, CO, and SVR
  g. Assess and document continuous ECG rhythm; vital signs; mental status;
     heart, lung, and bowel sounds; urine output; and any signs and
     symptoms indicating changes in these parameters
  h. Insert an NG tube to relieve gastric distention and prevent aspiration
  i. Administer antibiotics to treat the underlying infection
  j. Monitor and report any abnormalities in serum glucose and electrolyte
     levels
  k. Obtain ABG measurements and monitor for hypoxemia and acid-base
     imbalance
  l. Provide safety measures to prevent accidental injury from altered LOC
  m. Position the patient for comfort; elevate the head of the bed to facilitate
     respiration and prevent aspiration
  n. Teach the patient to recognize signs and symptoms of hyperglycemia
     requiring medical intervention
  o. Instruct the patient in the proper technique for blood glucose testing to
     monitor diabetes, and have him demonstrate the technique

E. Hypoglycemia
  1. General information
     a. Hypoglycemia is an emergency situation in which serum glucose levels decrease to less than 50 mg/dl
     b. Normal homeostatic mechanisms maintain serum glucose levels at 60 to 100 mg/dl
     c. Signs and symptoms appear suddenly and require immediate action to correct
     d. Hypoglycemia can occur as a rebound effect after high carbohydrate intake (known as the Somogyi phenomenon)
     e. Irreversible brain damage and myocardial infarction can occur if hypoglycemia is not promptly corrected
     f. Prompt reversal of hypoglycemia occurs with administration of concentrated glucose
  2. Possible causes
     a. Insulin overdose
     b. Inadequate carbohydrate intake
     c. Impaired glucose tolerance
     d. Extrapancreatic tumor
     e. Liver and adrenal insufficiency
     f. Medical therapy, such as gastric surgery
     g. Medications, such as sulfonylureas and beta blockers
  3. Assessment findings
     a. Cool, clammy skin
     b. Headache
     c. Diaphoresis
     d. Dizziness
     e. Staggering gait
     f. Hunger
     g. Nausea
     h. Agitation
     i. Fatigue
     j. Anxiety
     k. Tremors or seizures
     l. Blurred vision
     m. Inability to concentrate progressing to alteration in LOC
  4. Diagnostic test findings: Serum glucose levels below 50 mg/dl
  5. Patient care management goal: to elevate serum glucose levels promptly
     a. Administer 50% glucose I.V. over 2 to 5 minutes if the patient is unconscious
     b. Administer glucagon I.V. to stimulate liver glycogenolysis unless the patient has liver dysfunction
     c. Administer fluids I.V. for hydration and additional glucose for stabilization until oral intake is resumed

d. Give fast-acting carbohydrates, such as fruit juice, or sugar, honey, or corn syrup to relieve signs and symptoms if the patient is conscious

e. Follow with more complex carbohydrates, such as cheese and crackers, to stabilize serum glucose levels

f. When in doubt about the patient's glucose level (whether it is high or low), always give glucose

g. Protect the patient from injury that may result from confusion, seizures, or coma

h. Teach the patient signs and symptoms of hypoglycemia and proper measures to correct it

i. Instruct the patient about the proper technique for blood glucose testing, and have him demonstrate the technique

F. Syndrome of inappropriate antidiuretic hormone

1. General information
   a. Syndrome of inappropriate antidiuretic hormone is an endocrine dysfunction caused by uncontrolled production or excessive secretion of antidiuretic hormone (ADH)
   b. Normal ADH secretion is controlled by an increase in plasma osmolality, detection of decreased plasma volume in receptors located in the left atria and pulmonary vasculature, and detection of decreased blood pressure by carotid and aortic bodies
   c. Water is retained when ADH is secreted, and excessive secretion or production of ADH may result in water intoxication and cerebral edema
   d. As the kidneys attempt to compensate for the excess water, more sodium is filtered into the urine, causing severe hyponatremia

2. Causes
   a. Oat cell carcinoma of the lung
   b. Severe pneumonia
   c. Mechanical ventilation
   d. Other cancers, such as leukemia and cancers of the pancreas, prostate, and brain
   e. Head trauma
   f. Stress
   g. Medications, such as oral hypoglycemic agents, diuretics, and cytoxic agents

3. Assessment findings
   a. Weight gain without corresponding peripheral edema
   b. Decreased and concentrated urine
   c. Hypertension
   d. Elevated CVP, PAP, PAWP
   e. Nausea, vomiting, or diarrhea
   f. Anorexia
   g. Headache
   h. Altered LOC
   i. Seizure activity

4. Diagnostic test findings
   a. Serum sodium: less than 135 mEq/liter
   b. Serum osmolality: lower than urine osmolality
   c. Urine osmolality: higher than serum osmolality
   d. Urine specific gravity: greater than 1.030
   e. Plasma ADH: elevated
5. Patient care management goal: to correct the cause and restore the fluid and electrolyte balance
   a. Assess the fluid balance carefully; monitor intake and output; restrict fluids based on amounts lost in urine and as insensible losses
   b. Replace sodium losses with I.V. administration of hypertonic 3% saline solution
   c. Administer diuretic therapy to promote water excretion
   d. Administer demeclocycline and lithium to inhibit the action of ADH on the renal tubules and to promote water excretion
   e. Prepare the patient for pulmonary artery catheter placement to monitor fluid status and evaluate therapy
   f. Assess and document CVP, PAP, PAWP, CO, and SVR
   g. Assess and document continuous ECG rhythm; vital signs; mental status; heart, lung, and bowel sounds; urine output; and any signs and symptoms indicating changes in these parameters
   h. Monitor urine and serum diagnostic tests for abnormalities; ensure laboratory specimens are obtained correctly and expediently so that an accurate correlation can be made between fluid and medication administration
   i. Offer frequent mouth care and comfort measures when fluids are restricted
   j. Weigh the patient daily, at the same time and on the same scale, to evaluate fluid balance
   k. Prepare the patient for surgical intervention to remove the malignant lesion if it is the causative agent
   l. Teach the patient the importance of fluid restriction and daily weighing

G. Thyrotoxicosis (thyroid storm or crisis)
1. General information
   a. Thyrotoxicosis is a rapidly developing, life-threatening metabolic emergency caused by hyperthyroidism
   b. Excessive thyroid hormone produces an increased rate of all metabolic processes
   c. The mortality from thyrotoxicosis is greater than 20% if untreated
2. Causes
   a. Graves' disease
   b. Goiter or hyperfunctioning thyroid
   c. Excessive intake of exogenous thyroid hormone
   d. Abrupt cessation of antithyroid drugs

      e. Trauma
      f. Stress
      g. Infection
      h. DKA
      i. Toxemia of pregnancy

3. Assessment findings
      a. Heat intolerance
      b. Exophthalmos or dryness of eyes
      c. Enlarged thyroid gland
      d. Hyperthermia
      e. Dehydration
      f. Diaphoresis
      g. Flushing
      h. Tachycardia and tachypnea
      i. Nausea, vomiting, or diarrhea
      j. Weight loss
      k. Agitation or tremors

4. Diagnostic test findings
      a. Triiodothyronine (T_3) and thyroxine (T_4) levels: elevated
      b. Serum glucose: increased (from glycogenolysis or decreased insulin production or secretion)
      c. Serum calcium: elevated (from increased bone metabolism)
      d. Hb and HCT: elevated (from dehydration)
      e. ECG: tachycardia even during sleep, with frequently occurring premature atrial and ventricular beats and possibly atrial fibrillation

5. Patient care management goal: to support vital functions of the respiratory, cardiac, and renal systems and to reverse the peripheral effects of excessive thyroid hormone
      a. Maintain a patent airway; ensure the airway is not impaired by edema in the postoperative thyroidectomy patient
      b. Administer I.V. fluids for hydration and replacement of electrolytes
      c. Administer beta blockers to decrease the peripheral effects of thyroid hormone and to inhibit conversion of T_4 to T_3
      d. Administer propylthiouracil to inhibit conversion of T_4 to T_3
      e. Administer sodium or potassium iodide or Lugol's solution to inhibit release of iodine, which is essential for release of T_4 and T_3
      f. Administer glucocorticoids to block conversion of T_4 to T_3; this also may decrease adrenal insufficiency, which often accompanies thyroid storm
      g. Administer drug therapy to treat the underlying disease, such as DKA
      h. Prepare the patient for pulmonary artery catheter placement to monitor fluid status and evaluate therapy
      i. Assess and document CVP, PAP, PAWP, CO, and SVR
      j. Assess and document continuous ECG rhythm; vital signs; mental status; heart, lung, and bowel sounds; urine output; and any signs and symptoms indicating changes in these parameters

k. Maintain strict adherence to medication scheduling and dosing because drug conversion and degradation will be increased
l. Monitor T_3 and T_4 laboratory results, and report all abnormal values
m. Schedule activities to conserve the patient's energy
n. Provide a quiet room to decrease stimuli and reduce metabolic demands
o. Apply a cooling blanket for hyperthermia
p. Provide safety measures to prevent accidental injury from altered LOC, seizures, or coma
q. Avoid aspirin for fever control, because it replaces T_3 from carrier protein and increases free T_3 levels
r. Prepare the patient for surgical intervention to remove the malignant lesion if it is the causative agent
s. Teach the patient the importance of hormonal replacement therapy and strict compliance

Points to Remember

Fat breakdown for energy, in the absence of glucose, causes ketone formation.

Irreversible brain damage and myocardial infarction can occur if hypoglycemia is not promptly reversed.

When in doubt about glucose level, always give glucose; response will be immediate if the patient is hypoglycemic.

Strict adherence to medication schedules and doses is imperative for patients with endocrine dysfunction who may have abnormal drug turnover and degradation because of alterations in metabolism.

Glossary

Diabetes mellitus—condition produced by an alteration in glucose metabolism or use, causing the patient to be insulin-deficient

Exophthalmos—condition characterized by protrusion of the eyeballs, caused by hyperthyroidism

Glycogenolysis—process of breaking down glycogen into dextrose

Hormones—chemicals secreted by the endocrine glands that regulate metabolic functions

Ketonemia—ketones in blood

Polyphagia—excessive eating, a classic symptom of diabetes

Neurologic Disorders

Learning Objectives
After studying this section, the reader should be able to:

• Describe the general principles of neurologic function.

• Identify possible causes for each type of alteration in neurologic function.

• Discuss common assessment and diagnostic test findings for the patient with a specific alteration in neurologic function.

• Describe care management for the patient with a specific alteration in neurologic function.

XVI. Neurologic Disorders

A. Basic concepts

1. The nervous system directs all movement, sensation, emotion, and thought by its control over all other other body systems
2. Any interruption in the nervous system or in its blood supply can produce life-threatening effects
3. Signs and symptoms vary with the extent of injury and the area of brain involved
4. Potential nursing diagnoses for the patient with neurologic disorders may include:
   a. Altered tissue perfusion
   b. Sensory-perceptual alteration
   c. Ineffective airway clearance
   d. Potential for injury
   e. Altered comfort: pain
   f. Self-care deficit

B. Anatomy and physiology

1. The central nervous system (CNS) consists of the brain, brain stem, and spinal cord
   a. The *cerebrum* has two hemispheres; specialized areas of each hemisphere perform motor, sensory, mental, and associative functions
   b. The *diencephalon* consists of the hypothalamus (which affects water balance, appetite, temperature, emotion, pituitary secretions, and autonomic functions) and the thalamus (which helps control primitive responses, such as fear and self-preservation, and acts as a relay point for most afferent and efferent tracts)
   c. The *cerebellum* coordinates muscle movement with sensory input, controls balance, and maintains muscle tone
   d. The *brain stem* consists of the midbrain, pons, and medulla oblongata; it relays messages between the brain and lower levels of the nervous system
   e. Four *communicating ventricles* contain cerebrospinal fluid (CSF) and include two lateral ventricles and a third and fourth ventricle
   f. The *spinal cord* mediates the reflex arc and is the communicating pathway between the brain and the peripheral nervous system
2. The peripheral nervous system consists of the cranial and spinal nerves
   a. Cranial nerves: 12 pairs that primarily serve the motor and sensory needs of the head as well as those of the neck, chest, and abdomen
   b. Spinal nerves: 31 pairs, including 8 cervical, 12 thoracic, 5 lumbar, 5 sacral, and 1 coccygeal pair supplying upper and lower extremities
3. The brain receives about 20% of cardiac output, which provides a constant supply of oxygen and glucose to the brain cells
4. Sufficient cerebral blood flow is necessary to meet the metabolic needs of the brain and depends on an intact cerebrovascular system

5. Two compensatory mechanisms protect the brain under adverse conditions
   a. Collateral circulation allows for alternate blood flow if normal blood flow is occluded
   b. Autoregulation maintains constant blood flow through vasodilation or constriction stimulated by serum carbon dioxide and oxygen concentration and arterial blood pressure; autoregulation fails to function with mean arterial pressure less than 60 mm Hg or pathology associated with atherosclerosis, arterial rupture, or occlusion

C. **Cerebrovascular accident**
   1. General information
      a. Cerebrovascular accident (CVA) is a sudden, severe disruption of the blood supply to the brain, producing cerebral anoxia and alteration in cerebral metabolism
      b. CVA is classified as thrombotic or hemorrhagic
      c. *Thrombotic CVA* occurs when a cerebral artery is occluded by a thrombus or embolus
      d. *Hemorrhagic CVA* occurs from an intracerebral hemorrhage (ICH) or subarachnoid hemorrhage (SAH)
      e. CVA may also be categorized according to the side of the brain affected, either right or left.
      f. The signs and symptoms vary depending on the side of the brain affected
   2. Causes
      a. Thrombus
      b. Cerebral embolism
      c. Ruptured intracerebral artery, commonly from hypertension (ICH)
      d. Ruptured aneurysm or ruptured arteriovenous malformation (SAH)
   3. Assessment findings: left CVA
      a. Right hemiparesis or hemiplegia
      b. Right homonymous hemianopia
      c. Memory deficits in language
      d. Expressive or receptive aphasia
      e. Slow, cautious behavior
      f. Acute intellectual impairment
   4. Assessment findings: right CVA
      a. Left hemiparesis or hemiplegia
      b. Left homonymous hemianopia
      c. Memory deficits in performance
      d. Impulsive behavior
      e. Lack of motivation
      f. Spatial and perceptual deficits
   5. Diagnostic test findings
      a. Computed tomography (CT) scan: identifies the location and characteristics of a CVA, or the distortion or shift of ventricles with hemorrhage or edema

b. Magnetic resonance imaging: identifies changes in the cranial and spinal structures

c. Electroencephalogram (EEG): identifies seizure activity and changes in the brain's electrical waveforms

d. Angiography: identifies occlusion, stenosis, aneurysms, hemorrhage, and infarction of the arterial system

6. Patient care management goal: to support the patient's vital functions, restore cerebral blood flow, minimize neurologic deficits, and prevent progression

   a. Maintain a patent airway to promote adequate oxygenation

   b. Administer oxygen therapy with possible intubation and mechanical ventilation to ensure adequate tissue perfusion

   c. Maintain bed rest to minimize metabolic requirements

   d. Provide I.V. fluids to support blood pressure and maintain volume

   e. Administer dexamethasone to reduce cerebral edema

   f. Administer anticoagulants and antiplatelet drugs for thrombotic conditions after hemorrhage has been ruled out

   g. Administer sedatives, such as phenobarbital, to decrease metabolic requirements

   h. Assess the patient's neurologic status; observe for CVA progression and level of consciousness (LOC) changes as evidenced by decreasing numerical score on Glasgow Coma Scale

   i. Correct cardiovascular abnormalities, such as atrial fibrillation, that may be contributing factors

   j. Consider surgical procedures to correct circulatory impairment, prevent repeated hemorrhage, or relieve cerebral pressure

   k. Begin bedside range-of-motion exercises to preserve mobility and prevent deformities

   l. Teach the patient to identify risk factors and necessary life-style modifications, such as diet, stress reduction, and smoking cessation

   m. Direct the family to community groups that provide support or rehabilitation

D. Meningitis

1. General information

   a. Meningitis is an inflammation of the brain and spinal cord that may involve all meningeal membranes

   b. Meningitis is classified as bacterial, fungal, or viral

   c. *Bacterial meningitis* is commonly a complication of bacteremia

   d. *Fungal meningitis* is caused by fungal infections of the CNS

   e. *Viral meningitis* occurs as a complication of systemic viral infections

   f. The most common type of meningitis is bacterial, a medical emergency that may be fatal within a few days if not treated

   g. Prompt recognition of the causative organism ensures the best prognosis

ASSESSING LEVEL OF CONSCIOUSNESS USING THE GLASGOW COMA SCALE

To assess a patient's level of consciousness quickly in an emergency, use the Glasgow Coma Scale. Below is an expanded version of this useful—though not comprehensive—assessment technique. (A patient scoring 7 or less is comatose and probably has severe neurologic damage.)

TEST	SCORE	PATIENT'S RESPONSE
Verbal response (when you ask, "What year is this?")		
Oriented	5	He tells you the current year.
Confused	4	He tells you an incorrect year.
Inappropriate words	3	He replies randomly: "tomorrow" or "roses."
Incomprehensible	2	He moans or screams.
None	1	He gives no response.
Eye opening response		
Spontaneously	4	He opens his eyes spontaneously.
To speech	3	He opens his eyes when you tell him to.
To pain	2	He opens his eyes only on painful stimulus (for example, application of pressure to bony ridge under eyebrow).
None	1	He doesn't open his eyes in response to any stimulus.
Motor response		
Obeys	6	He shows you two fingers when you ask him to.
Localizes	5	He reaches toward the painful stimulation and tries to remove it.
Withdraws	4	He moves away from a painful stimulus.
Abnormal flexion	3	He assumes a decorticate posture (below).

Abnormal extension	2	He assumes a decerebrate posture (below).

None	1	He doesn't respond at all, just lies flaccid—an ominous sign.

     h. Permanent secondary damage and death can occur from the cerebral edema associated with the inflammation

     i. Prevalence of meningitis increases in people who live in crowded conditions and those in contact with farm animals, ticks, or fleas

2. Causes: bacterial meningitis
   a. Otitis media
   b. Respiratory infection or sinusitis
   c. Bacteremia
   d. Immunologic reactions
   e. Metastatic infections

3. Causes: fungal meningitis
   a. Complication of acquired immunodeficiency syndrome
   b. Histoplasmosis
   c. Contaminated needles or syringes from drug abuse

4. Causes: viral meningitis
   a. Enteroviruses
   b. Mumps
   c. Herpes simplex
   d. Chicken pox
   e. Arbovirus

5. Assessment findings: bacterial meningitis
   a. Nuchal rigidity
   b. Chills
   c. Fever
   d. Lethargy
   e. Positive Brudzinski's and Kernig's signs
   f. Nausea and vomiting
   g. Headache
   h. Generalized seizures

6. Assessment findings: fungal meningitis
   a. Headache
   b. Fever
   c. Personality changes
   d. Positive Brudzinski's and Kernig's signs

7. Assessment findings: viral meningitis
   a. Headache
   b. Pain when moving the eyes
   c. Weakness
   d. Painful extremities
   e. Positive Brudzinski's and Kernig's signs

8. Diagnostic test findings
   a. Lumbar puncture: identifies the type of causative agent by abnormality of glucose, protein, and white blood cell (WBC) count
   b. Blood cultures: positive for causative organism
   c. Counter immunoelectrophoresis: bacterial antigens in CSF and urine
   d. WBC count: elevated in presence of infection

9. Patient care management goal: to diagnose and treat the condition promptly
    a. Maintain a patent airway and provide supplemental oxygen as prescribed
    b. Use isolation precautions based on Centers for Disease Control guidelines and institutional policy; bacterial meningitis is transmitted through droplets or contact with oral secretions; viral meningitis is transmitted through contact with stool and oral secretions; fungal meningitis is transmitted through the air and blood stream
    c. Provide for patient safety and anticonvulsant therapy if seizure activity is present
    d. Assess the patient's nutritional status; institute measures to maintain adequate nutrition
    e. Administer antibiotic and antifungal therapy determined by the causative organism (viral meningitis requires no drug therapy), and document the patient's response to therapy
    f. Observe for signs and symptoms of increased intracranial pressure (ICP), such as headaches, vomiting, fluctuations in heart rate and blood pressure, and widening pulse pressure
    g. Monitor the patient to be sure he avoids activities that increase ICP, such as straining, coughing, and bending; make sure he understands the importance of avoiding these activities
    h. Use a cooling blanket, antipyretics, and tepid baths to maintain the patient's temperature within the prescribed range
    i. Direct the family to community groups that provide support or rehabilitation

E. Drug overdose

1. General information
    a. Drug overdose occurs when a drug is ingested in amounts greater than recommended, which produces alterations in the neurologic, respiratory, or cardiac systems; overdose may be accidental or intentional
    b. Drug overdose is a widespread problem that affects people of all ages, races, and socioeconomic groups
    c. Emergency department staff must be thoroughly knowledgeable about the treatments and complications of overdose to ensure patient survival
    d. Prognosis is based on the type and amount of drug ingested and the speed of medical intervention
    e. Patients may minimize or exaggerate the amount of drug ingested
    f. The effects of injected substances, such as heroin or narcotics, can be reversed with an antidote (Narcan)
    g. The effects of ingested substances can be treated with induced emesis, gastric lavage, or adsorption
    h. Ipecac syrup is the safest and most effective means to induce emesis; home remedies may be unsafe and ineffective; a gag reflex must be present, and LOC should not be depressed when administering the syrup, or aspiration may occur

      i.   All persons who intentionally overdose should be referred for psychiatric evaluation before discharge

      j.   The patient may repeat a suicide attempt while hospitalized

2.   Causes

    a.   Suicidal or attention-seeking gesture

    b.   Accidental ingestion of drugs, primarily by children

    c.   Knowledge deficit regarding dosing of prescribed drug

3.   Assessment findings: signs and symptoms vary with the type and amount of drug ingested; life-threatening findings include:

    a.   Respiratory arrest

    b.   Cardiac dysrhythmias or conduction disturbance

    c.   Seizures

    d.   Cardiovascular collapse

    e.   Coma

4.   Diagnostic test findings

    a.   Drug toxicology screen of serum and urine: positive for presence and type of drug

    b.   Serum alcohol: positive for presence and amount of alcohol

    c.   CT scan: rules out other pathologic conditions

    d.   Lumbar puncture: rules out other pathologic conditions

    e.   ECG: normal or reveals cardiac dysrhythmias

5.   Patient care management goal: to stabilize the patient, identify the drug, reverse its effects, and eliminate it from the patient's body

    a.   Maintain a patent airway and provide supplemental oxygen and respiratory support, as indicated

    b.   Induce vomiting (if the patient is conscious) or perform gastric lavage to reverse or eliminate the toxic substance; document the patient's response (give no more than two doses of Ipecac Syrup; perform gastric lavage until the return is clear; do not give Ipecac and activated charcoal together because the charcoal inactivates the Ipecac)

    c.   Provide continuous cardiac monitoring because many drugs cause cardiac dysrhythmias

    d.   Evaluate the patient's LOC, using the Glasgow coma scale

    e.   Provide suicide precautions and psychiatric evaluation, as necessary

    f.   Consider hemodialysis if toxic substance levels require immediate elimination

    g.   Administer anticonvulsive therapy, as indicated, to minimize or prevent seizure activity

    h.   If restraints are necessary, place the patient on his side to prevent aspiration

    i.   Depending on the situation, teach the patient measures to prevent accidental poisonings, refer him for counseling to prevent intentional overdoses, or provide accurate drug dose information to ensure that he is taking necessary medications correctly

      j. Refer the patient and family to community resources that can provide support

      k. Be sure the patient and family know the telephone number of the nearest poison control center or crisis hot line

F. Status epilepticus

1. General information
   a. Status epilepticus is acute, prolonged seizure activity that occurs without full recovery of consciousness between convulsions
   b. Status epilepticus is a medical emergency because the constant activity may deplete the brain of oxygen and glucose, which may produce hypoxia and neuronal death

2. Causes
   a. Noncompliance with medication treatment
   b. Concurrent infection
   c. Alcohol abuse
   d. Fever

3. Assessment findings
   a. Alteration in LOC
   b. Tonic or clonic body movements
   c. Incontinence of urine or stool
   d. Automatisms: involuntary motor activities, such as lip smacking, swallowing, or chewing

4. Diagnostic test findings
   a. Serum chemistries: metabolic or electrolyte imbalance
   b. Serum alcohol: positive for presence and quantity of alcohol
   c. EEG: negative for other pathologic conditions
   d. CT scan: negative for other pathologic conditions
   e. Anticonvulsant serum drug levels: subtherapeutic or therapeutic amount of drug in blood

5. Patient care management goal: to ensure adequate cerebral oxygenation and to stop seizure activity
   a. Maintain a patent airway and adequate oxygenation, with possible intubation
   b. Administer short-term anticonvulsant therapy, such as diazepam, until the patient is seizure-free
   c. Administer long-acting anticonvulsant therapy, such as phenytoin or phenobarbital; infuse phenytoin I.V. with normal saline solution only, to prevent a reaction with dextrose-containing solutions
   d. Consider general anesthesia or neuromuscular blocking agents to stop seizure activity if other anticonvulsants are unsuccessful
   e. Protect the patient during seizure activity: avoid restraining him or forcing anything through clenched teeth; move potentially dangerous items away from him
   f. Keep the patient turned to the side during the seizure to prevent aspiration

g. Monitor and document duration of seizure activity, any associated signs, and the patient's LOC after seizure activity

h. Reassure the patient when he awakens to alleviate his anxiety

i. Document the name of the drug, the last dose, and the medication regimen if the patient is taking anticonvulsant medications

j. Teach the patient and family the importance of complying with treatment, activating the emergency medical system if needed, and having the patient wear a Medic Alert bracelet if the seizure disorder is chronic

G. Myasthenic crisis

1. General information

   a. Myasthenic crisis is the sudden onset of weakness in the patient with myasthenia gravis, often manifested by sudden respiratory distress or the inability to speak or swallow

   b. Myasthenia gravis is an autoimmune disease in which antibodies attack the acetylcholine receptor sites at the postsynaptic membrane, impairing neuromuscular transmission

   c. Progressive weakness of the diaphragm and intercostal muscles is a medical emergency because it may lead to respiratory failure

   d. The patient with myasthenia gravis may develop other crises in response to drug therapy

   e. *Cholinergic crisis* may occur from overmedication with anticholinesterase drugs

   f. *Brittle crisis* may occur from desensitivity of receptors at the neuromuscular junction to anticholinesterase drugs

   g. The patient with myasthenia gravis should recognize the risk factors that precipitate myasthenic crisis, such as emotional stress, systemic infections, and exposure to heat or cold

2. Causes

   a. Progression of the disease

   b. Systemic infections

   c. Emotional stress

   d. Surgery

   e. Trauma

   f. Certain drugs, such as morphine, beta blockers, some anticonvulsants, cardiac drugs, and antibiotics

   g. Exposure to heat or cold

3. Assessment findings

   a. Decrease in chest expansion and air movement

   b. Weakness of the ocular, respiratory, and bulbar muscles

   c. Increased anxiety

   d. Dysphagia

   e. Dysarthria

   f. Ptosis of eyelids

   g. Diplopia

4. Diagnostic test findings: signs and symptoms may be so significant for myasthenia gravis that diagnosis may be made on the basis of history and physical examination
   a. Tensilon test: muscle weakness and fatigue decrease within 1 minute; the improvement lasts for up to 5 minutes after I.V. administration of edrophonium chloride (Tensilon)
   b. Neostigmine bromide test: muscle weakness and fatigue improve within 15 minutes and last for up to 2 hours after I.M. administration of neostigmine
   c. Electromyography: rapid decrease in the amplitude of evoked potentials
   d. Serum antibodies against acetylcholine receptor (antiAChR antibodies): positive
5. Patient care management goal: to provide respiratory support, preserve remaining muscle function, and reduce and remove circulating antibodies
   a. Maintain a patent airway, provide supplemental oxygen, and consider mechanical respiratory support, if necessary
   b. Administer anticholinesterase drugs, such as neostigmine, to increase the availability of acetylcholine at the neuromuscular junction
   c. Begin immunosuppressive therapy, such as administering corticosteroids, using plasmapheresis, or preparing for thymectomy
   d. Assess the patient for the presence of a gag reflex and the ability to swallow
   e. Administer medications at the exact times ordered; delay in administration time, may result in difficulty in swallowing
   f. Place the patient in a sitting position with his neck slightly flexed to aid swallowing
   g. Determine effective ways to communicate with the patient so his needs are met
   h. Administer artificial tears to protect corneas in the patient with ptosis
   i. Teach the patient and family the importance of taking medications at the prescribed times; be sure they know risk factors and can recognize signs and symptoms warranting medical attention, such as respiratory distress, ptosis, diplopia, or dysphasia

H. Increased intracranial pressure
1. General information
   a. Increased intracranial pressure (ICP) is an elevation of the pressure exerted within the skull by the intracranial volume above 15 mm Hg
   b. Increased ICP is not a disease but the result of conditions that alter intracranial volume
   c. When ICP increases to pathologic levels, brain damage can occur because the rigid skull allows little space for expansion
   d. The brain compensates for increases in ICP by regulating the intracranial volume (limiting blood flow to the head), displacing CSF into the spinal canal, and increasing or decreasing CSF production

e. When compensatory mechanisms become overworked, small changes in intracranial volume lead to large changes in ICP

f. Hypercarbia and hypoxia contribute to changes in ICP because they cause cerebral vasodilation, which in turn increases blood volume and ICP

PATHOPHYSIOLOGY OF INCREASED INTRACRANIAL PRESSURE

Brain insult

↓

Slight increase in intracranial pressure (ICP)

↓

Attempt at normal regulation of ICP by decreased blood flow to head

↓

Slight decrease in cerebral perfusion pressure (CPP)

↓

Loss of autoregulatory mechanism of constriction or dilation of cerebral blood vessels if increased ICP persists

↓

Passive dilation

↓

Increased cerebral blood flow; venous congestion

↓

Further increase in ICP

↓

Uncal or central herniation

↓

Further decrease in CPP

↓

Cellular hypoxia

↓

Brain death

2. Causes
   a. Head injuries
   b. Aneurysms
   c. CVA
   d. Brain tumors
   e. Reye's syndrome
   f. Impaired autoregulation
   g. Hydrocephalus
3. Assessment findings
   a. Deteriorating LOC
   b. Pupillary dilation
   c. Decreased pupillary light reflex
   d. Loss of motor function
   e. Sensory deterioration
   f. Vital sign changes
   g. Vomiting
4. Diagnostic test findings
   a. CT scan: cerebral structure shifts from tumor, hematomas, and hydrocephalus
   b. Brain scan: cerebral hemorrhage, hematoma, or tumor
   c. ICP monitoring: increased ICP
5. Patient care management goal: to reduce ICP, improve cerebral perfusion pressure (CPP), and decrease brain tissue distortion
   a. Maintain a patent airway; intubate and mechanically ventilate to prevent hypoxia and hypercarbia
   b. Consider surgery to remove intracranial masses
   c. Administer osmotic agents, such as mannitol or urea, to decrease CSF volume and increase CPP
   d. Consider diuretics, such as furosemide, to decrease CSF volume
   e. Administer steroids, such as dexamethasone, to reduce brain edema and ICP
   f. Drain CSF, if a ventricular drainage system is in place, based on the doctor's order and the patient's condition
   g. Consider administering barbiturates, such as phenobarbital, to induce coma if the patient is refractory to other therapy (use is contrversial because of the potential complication of hypotension, which may further alter the CPP)
   h. Use the Glasgow Coma Scale and the institution's neurologic flow sheet to assess changes in LOC
   i. Monitor ABG measurements to prevent hypoxia and hypercapnia

j. Maintain partial pressures of carbon dioxide in arterial blood between 25 to 35 mm Hg to prevent cerebral vasodilation produced by hypercapnia

k. Keep partial pressures of oxygen in arterial blood within normal limits to prevent cerebral vasodilation produced by hypoxia

l. Preoxygenate and hyperventilate before and after suctioning to prevent hypoxia

m. Limit suctioning to 10 to 15 seconds to prevent hypoxia

n. Elevate the head of the bed 15 to 30 degrees, or as ordered, to facilitate venous return

o. Avoid neck rotation, flexion, or extension to facilitate venous return

p. If a tracheostomy or endotracheal tube is required, make sure ties are not too tight to impede venous return

q. Space out activities known to increase ICP, such as suctioning, turning, and Valsalva's maneuver

Points to Remember

Autoregulation is maintained in the brain by vasodilation or constriction and serum O_2 and CO_2 levels.

The Glasgow coma scale is an objective way to measure LOC.

Bacterial meningitis is the most common type of meningitis. Signs of meningeal irritation include nuchal rigidity and positive Brudzinski's and Kernig's signs.

All patients who intentionally overdose should be referred for psychiatric evaluation before discharge from the hospital.

Small changes in intracranial volume lead to large changes in ICP.

Glossary

Brudzinski's sign—assessment technique used to determine the presence of meningitis; it is considered positive when forward flexion of the neck causes hip and knee flexion

Dysarthria—difficulty in speaking caused by impairment of innervated speech organs

Glasgow Coma Scale—assessment tool that evaluates the patient's level of consciousness according to three categories: eye opening, motor response, and verbal response

Kernig's sign—assessment technique used to determine the presence of meningitis; it is considered positive when attempts to flex the hip of a recumbent person produce painful spasms of the hamstring muscle and resistance to further leg extension at the knee

Ptosis—abnormal drooping of the upper eyelid

Gastrointestinal Disorders

Learning Objectives
After studying this section, the reader should be able to:

• Describe the general principles of gastrointestinal (GI) system function.

• Identify possible causes for each type of alteration in GI function.

• Discuss common assessment and diagnostic test findings for the patient with a specific GI disorder.

• Describe care management for the patient with a specific alteration in GI function.

XVII. Gastrointestinal Disorders

A. Basic concepts

1. The GI system is also called the alimentary tract or the digestive system
   a. Begins at the mouth
   b. Ends at the anus
2. The GI system functions to mechanically and chemically alter ingested food so that nutritional needs are met
3. Potential nursing diagnoses for the patient with GI dysfunction include:
   a. Altered nutrition
   b. Fluid volume deficit
   c. Altered bowel elimination
   d. Altered tissue perfusion
   e. Anxiety
   f. Altered comfort: pain

B. Anatomy and physiology

1. The GI system consists of the:
   a. Mouth
   b. Esophagus
   c. Stomach
   d. Small intestine
   e. Large intestine
2. Four accessory organs aid the digestive system
   a. Salivary glands
   b. Pancreas
   c. Gallbladder
   d. Liver
3. The arterial blood supply to the GI tract is primarily delivered through the mesenteric arteries
4. The portal venous system collects and delivers venous blood from the GI tract to the liver and eventually back into the inferior vena cava
5. The GI tract is under control of the autonomic nervous system

C. Acute GI bleeding: Ulcer

1. General information
   a. Acute GI bleeding is a life-threatening emergency caused by ulceration of the GI mucosa and characterized by gross vomiting or defecation of occult stool
   b. Upper GI hemorrhage is produced from any site proximal to the cecum and includes ulcers of the mouth, stomach, or duodenum, or gastritis or esophageal varices
   c. Peptic ulcer disease includes duodenal or gastric ulcers
   d. Most ulcers are duodenal and occur in middle age
   e. Gastric ulcers, occurring after age 50, are likely to become malignant

    f. Lower GI hemorrhage is produced from any site distal to the cecum and includes ruptured diverticuli and ischemic bowel polyps, tumors, or eroding aortic aneurysm

    g. Ulcerative erosion occurs from excess hydrochloric acid (HCl)

    h. Most acute GI bleeding is from an arterial source

    i. Estimated blood loss is an index to the severity of the bleeding

    j. A blood loss greater than 20% causes decreased venous return and cardiac output

2. Causes
   a. Stress
   b. Trauma, including surgery
   c. Burns
   d. Drugs that stimulate HCl release, such as reserpine
   e. Drugs that decrease blood supply to the GI tract, such as vasopressors
   f. Drugs that alter mucosal integrity, such as aspirin, anticoagulants, and steroids
   g. Stimulants, such as nicotine and caffeine
   h. Biliary or pancreatic disease

3. Assessment findings
   a. Hematemesis
   b. Melena (black, tarlike stool)
   c. Hematochezia (bloody stool)
   d. Diarrhea
   e. Mild to severe abdominal pain
   f. Weakness
   g. Dysphagia or heartburn
   h. Signs of shock, including hypotension, tachycardia, diaphoresis, pallor, and decreased urine output

4. Diagnostic test findings
   a. Stool guaiac: positive
   b. Emesis guaiac: positive
   c. Hemoglobin (Hb) and hematocrit (HCT): decreased
   d. Arterial blood gas (ABG) measurements: acidosis if shock is present, causing lactic acidosis
   e. ECG: ischemic changes if hypoperfusion exists
   f. Endoscopy: source of the bleeding
   g. Biopsy: if cancer is the source of the bleeding
   h. Upper and lower GI tract X-rays: air and contrast (barium) indicating area of bleeding

5. Patient care management goal: to control shock and bleeding
   a. Maintain a patent airway to prevent aspiration of emesis or blood
   b. Administer oxygen therapy to treat hypoxia from a decrease in Hb
   c. Administer I.V. fluids, both crystalloids (such as lactated Ringer's solution) and colloids (such as plasmanate and blood), for volume expansion

    d. Insert a nasogastric (NG) tube for lavage with iced saline or water to decrease or control bleeding

    e. Administer antacids to raise pH, thus decreasing acidity

    f. Administer histamine$_2$ (H$_2$) receptor antagonist, such as cimetidine or ranitidine, to decrease gastric acid production

    g. Administer vasopressin for massive bleeding

    h. Provide parenteral nutrition to support the patient's metabolic needs

    i. Prepare the patient for pulmonary artery catheter placement to monitor fluid status and evaluate therapy

    j. Assess and document central venous pressure (CVP), pulmonary artery pressure (PAP), pulmonary artery wedge pressure (PAWP), cardiac output (CO), and systemic vascular resistance (SVR) as ordered

    k. Assess and document continuous ECG rhythm; vital signs; mental status; heart, lung, and bowel sounds; urine output; and any signs and symptoms indicating changes in these parameters

    l. Measure and record all fluid losses from the GI tract

    m. Check all emesis, stool, and drainage for blood

    n. Monitor Hb and HCT results, and report all abnormal values

    o. Provide comfort measures, such as oral care, and remove all soiled and odorous materials on or near the bed

    p. Provide emotional support to decrease fear and anxiety

    q. Prevent transmission of infection by washing hands thoroughly and wearing gloves when contact with blood or body fluids is likely to occur

    r. Prepare the patient for surgical intervention for ligation of bleeding vessels or removal of the ulcer or malignant lesion

    s. Teach the patient the importance of seeking medical attention if signs and symptoms of bleeding recur

D. Acute pancreatitis

  1. General information

    a. Pancreatitis is an inflammatory disease of the pancreas caused by an autodigestive process of pancreatic tissue by its own enzymes

    b. Trypsin is the enzyme responsible for initiating autodigestion

    c. The pancreas functions normally before and after an acute pancreatic episode

    d. Necrosis and hemorrhage are precursors of complete pancreatic dysfunction

    e. Mortality from pancreatitis may be greater than 70% in patients with necrosis and hemorrhage

    f. Respiratory failure is a common complication because the pancreas releases phospholipase, which destroys surfactant

    g. Other potential life-threatening complications include intravascular coagulopathies, renal failure, circulatory collapse, and sepsis

2. Causes
   a. Excessive alcohol intake (causes over 60% of cases)
   b. Hyperlipidemia
   c. Certain drugs, including corticosteroids, thiazide diuretics, and estrogens
   d. Biliary tract dysfunction with reflux or stones
   e. Viral or bacterial infection
   f. Trauma
   g. Surgical procedures involving the gastric, biliary, and cardiac organs
3. Assessment findings
   a. Epigastric pain, often radiating to the back
   b. Nausea, vomiting, or diarrhea
   c. Fever
   d. Abdominal rigidity
   e. Jaundice
   f. Hypotension
   g. Hypoventilation with crackles
   h. Positive Chvostek's and Trousseau's signs if hypocalcemia is present
4. Diagnostic test findings
   a. Serum amylase: elevated
   b. Urine amylase: elevated
   c. Serum glucose: elevated
   d. Serum calcium: decreased
   e. White blood cell (WBC) count: elevated count indicates inflammation
   f. Coagulation studies: decrease in platelets and fibrin
   g. Hb and HCT: decreased if bleeding
   h. Abdominal X-ray: calcification in epigastric area if process is chronic
   i. ABG measurements: hypoxemia and respiratory alkalosis initially, then acidosis as the patient's condition deteriorates
   j. ECG: ST and T-wave abnormalities from hypoxia and widening ST from hypocalcemia
5. Patient care management goal: to relieve pain, to rest the pancreas by minimizing demands for insulin and enzymes, and to maintain adequate circulating fluid volume
   a. Administer oxygen therapy if hypoxia is present
   b. Intubate and mechanically ventilate if the patient cannot maintain breathing
   c. Administer meperidine hydrochloride for pain rather than morphine, which can cause spasms of pancreatic and biliary ducts
   d. Administer I.V. fluids for hydration, volume expansion, and electrolyte replacement
   e. Administer insulin if hyperglycemia is present
   f. Insert an NG tube to relieve gastric distention and suppress pancreatic secretion
   g. Prepare the patient for pulmonary artery catheter placement to monitor fluid status and evaluate therapy
   h. Assess and document CVP, PAP, PAWP, CO, and SVR, as ordered

i. Assess and document continuous ECG rhythm; vital signs; mental status; heart, lung, and bowel sounds; urine output; and any signs and symptoms indicating changes in these parameters

j. Provide parenteral nutrition to support metabolic needs and defend against infection

k. Administer antibiotics appropriate for the causative organism

l. Limit activity to decrease metabolic demands

m. Measure and record all fluid losses from the GI tract

n. Monitor serum glucose and amylase levels, and report all abnormal values

o. Offer frequent mouth care and comfort measures when fluids are restricted or an NG tube is in place

p. Prevent transmission of infection by washing hands thoroughly and wearing gloves when contact with blood or body fluids is likely

q. Provide emotional support to decrease fear and anxiety

r. Teach the patient the importance of avoiding alcohol if it is a causative factor

E. Hepatic failure

1. General information

a. Hepatic (liver) failure is loss of normal liver functions because of damage to and destruction of hepatocytes

b. Liver functions are complex chemical processes that include vascular control, secretory function, metabolic regulation, and storage of reserve nutrients

c. In hepatic failure, liver cells are progressively destroyed and replaced with fibrotic tissue

d. Nearly 75% of liver tissue can be destroyed without the patient having signs and symptoms

e. Liver cells can regenerate and potentially reverse cellular damage if the patient survives the acute attack

2. Causes

a. Alcoholic or Laennec's cirrhosis

b. GI bleeding

c. Stress

d. Hypovolemia from shock or rapid diuresis

e. Infection

f. Hepatotoxic drugs, such as halothane, isoniazid, and acetaminophen

g. Type B and type non-A, non-B hepatitis

h. Obstructive biliary disease

3. Assessment findings

a. Jaundice

b. Anorexia or weight loss

c. Altered level of consciousness (LOC) progressing to coma

d. Asterixis

e. Ascites or edema

   f.   Dyspnea or decreased breath sounds
   g.   Ecchymosis, purpura, and bleeding from the oral mucosa
   h.   Fever
   i.   Hypertension
   j.   Increased CO associated with decreased SVR initially, then progressing
        to shock
   k.   Fetor hepaticus (fecal odor to breath)
   l.   Rectal and esophageal varices
   m.   Endocrine changes, such as testicular atrophy and gynecomastia in males
        and erratic menses in females
4.   Diagnostic test findings
   a.   Serum ammonia: elevated because of inability to convert to urea
   b.   Serum alkaline phosphatase: elevated because of inability to excrete
   c.   Blood urea nitrogen (BUN): increased because of renal failure or
        bleeding
   d.   Serum bilirubin: elevated because of failure in hepatocyte metabolism;
        may indicate poor prognosis
   e.   Serum albumin: decreased and may indicate poor prognosis
   f.   Complete blood count (CBC): decreased Hb, HCT, red blood cell (RBC)
        count; may reflect bleeding
   g.   Prothrombin time (PT): prolonged because of decrease in synthesis of
        vitamin K clotting factors
   h.   WBC count: elevated with infection
   i.   Hepatitis B surface antigen (HB_sAg) screen: detects active hepatitis
   j.   Liver biopsy: may determine cause of dysfunction
5.   Patient care management goal: to correct the causative factors and prevent
     further damage and complications
   a.   Administer oxygen to correct hypoxia
   b.   Administer I.V. fluids for hydration, volume expansion, and electrolyte
        replacement
   c.   Administer packed RBCs if needed for decreased HCT
   d.   Administer fresh frozen plasma if needed for clotting factors
   e.   Prepare the patient for pulmonary artery catheter placement to monitor
        fluid status and evaluate therapy
   f.   Assess and document CVP, PAP, PAWP, CO, and SVR as ordered
   g.   Assess and document continuous ECG rhythm; vital signs; mental status;
        heart, lung, and bowel sounds; urine output; and any signs and
        symptoms indicating changes in these parameters
   h.   Insert an NG tube to relieve gastric distention and to administer
        medications
   i.   Administer thiamine replacement if the patient is an alcoholic or
        thiamine levels are deficient
   j.   Administer H_2 receptor antagonist to prevent gastric erosion from stress
   k.   Administer neomycin to reduce ammonia-producing bacteria in the bowel
   l.   Administer lactulose to induce osmotic diarrhea

m. Administer parenteral nutrition, including a high-calorie, low-protein, low-sodium diet, if the GI tract is nonfunctional

n. Monitor serum albumin, alkaline phosphatase, BUN, bilirubin, and laboratory results, and report all abnormal values

o. Offer frequent mouth care and comfort measures when fluids are restricted

p. Institute protective measures to prevent skin damage, including lotion, pressure-relief devices, and position changes

q. Provide safety measures to prevent accidental injury from altered LOC, seizures, or coma

r. Prevent transmission of infection by washing hands thoroughly and wearing gloves when contact with blood or body fluids is likely

s. Prepare the patient for paracentesis, ultrafiltration, or peritoneal venous shunt to remove ascites

t. Prepare the patient for surgical intervention, including hepatic resection or transplant

u. Provide emotional support to decrease fear and anxiety

v. Teach the patient the importance of avoiding alcohol if it is a causative factor

F. Bleeding esophageal varices

1. General information
   a. Bleeding esophageal varices are varicose veins in the esophagus that have ruptured
   b. Portal hypertension with pressures elevated from the normal 8 to 12 mm Hg to over 30 mm Hg causes hypertrophy of veins and risk of rupture
   c. Varices most commonly occur in the distal esophagus
   d. The mortality from bleeding esophageal varices may be as high as 60% with the first episode
   e. Rebleeding with an even higher mortality rate is likely within the first year

2. Causes
   a. Cirrhosis
   b. Hepatitis
   c. Biliary infection
   d. Biliary disease, including stones or tumor
   e. Trauma, including surgery to portal venous system

3. Assessment findings
   a. Sudden and painless hematemesis
   b. Hypovolemia from blood loss
   c. Melena
   d. Other signs and symptoms of GI bleeding or hepatic failure (see "Acute GI bleeding: Ulcer," item C, and "Hepatic failure," item E, in this section)

4. Diagnostic test findings
   a. CBC: decreased Hb, HCT, platelet count
   b. Liver function studies (lactate dehydrogenase, serum glutamic-oxaloacetic transaminase, serum glutamic-pyruvic transaminase): elevated
   c. BUN: increased
   d. PT: prolonged
   e. Endoscopy: visualizes and localizes source of bleeding
5. Patient care management goal: to control the bleeding and prevent complications of shock and further liver failure
   a. Administer oxygen if hypoxia is present
   b. Intubate and mechanically ventilate if the patient cannot maintain breathing
   c. Administer vasopressin to constrict mesenteric, splenic, and hepatic arterioles and to decrease blood flow to portal system
   d. Administer nitroprusside or nitroglycerin, if required, to decrease peripheral vasoconstriction
   e. Prepare the patient for balloon tamponade with such devices as a Sengstaken-Blakemore, Minnesota, or Linton tube to temporarily control bleeding
   f. Maintain balloon tamponade by using adequate pressure inflation and deflation, as ordered, to prevent tissue necrosis from excessive pressure
   g. Keep scissors at bedside for prompt cutting and removal of balloon tamponade if gastric balloon ruptures and tube rises to occlude airway
   h. Administer I.V. fluids for hydration and volume expansion to replace losses
   i. Avoid using saline solutions, which contribute to ascites and edema
   j. Prepare the patient for pulmonary artery catheter placement to monitor fluid status and evaluate therapy
   k. Assess and document CVP, PAP, PAWP, CO, and SVR
   l. Assess and document continuous ECG rhythm; vital signs; mental status; heart, lung, and bowel sounds; urine output; and any signs and symptoms indicating changes in these parameters
   m. Prepare the patient for sclerotherapy (dilated varices are injected with a sclerosing agent, causing fibrosis) to control bleeding
   n. Monitor Hb and HCT, and report all abnormal results
   o. Measure and record all losses from bleeding
   p. Administer parenteral nutrition to support the patient's metabolic needs and defend against infection
   q. Prevent transmission of infection by washing hands thoroughly and wearing gloves when contact with blood or body fluids is likely
   r. Offer frequent mouth care and comfort measures when fluids are restricted
   s. Provide emotional support to decrease fear and anxiety
   t. Prepare the patient for possible implantation of a portacaval shunt to reduce portal hypertension

Points to Remember

Most acute GI bleeding is from an arterial source.

All emesis, stool, and drainage of patients with acute GI bleeding should be checked for blood.

GI pain in acute pancreatitis should be treated with meperidine rather than morphine, which can cause spasms of the pancreatic and biliary ducts.

Transmission of infection can be prevented by washing hands thoroughly and wearing gloves when contact with blood or body fluids is likely.

Glossary

Asterixis—flapping tremor of hands with finger flexion

Balloon tamponade—catheter device with a balloon that, when inflated, exerts pressure on bleeding varices in the esophagus or stomach

Guaiac test—test to determine the presence of blood; it uses a reagent solution that turns blue when blood is present

Jaundice—yellow skin color that occurs because of elevated serum bilirubin levels

Melena—black, tarlike stool

Female Reproductive Disorders

Learning Objectives

After studying this section, the reader should be able to:

● Describe the general principles of reproductive complications.

● Identify possible causes for each type of alteration in reproductive function.

● Discuss common assessment and diagnostic test findings for the patient with a specific alteration in reproductive function.

● Describe care management for the patient with a specific alteration in reproductive function.

XVIII. Female Reproductive Disorders

A. Basic concepts

1. Reproductive emergencies risk the health and life of both the mother and the fetus
2. The emergency department nurse is likely to see the woman with reproductive risks at admission; depending on the institution, complicated pregnancies may be cared for on the obstetric floor or in the intensive care unit
3. Potential nursing diagnoses for the patient with a reproductive disorder include:
   a. Anticipatory or dysfunctional grieving
   b. Altered cardiac output: decreased
   c. Altered comfort: pain
   d. Potential for injury

B. Anatomy and physiology

1. The female reproductive system includes the breasts and external and internal genital organs
2. The external genital organs include:
   a. Mons pubis
   b. Labia majora
   c. Labia minora
   d. Clitoris
   e. Vaginal vestibule
   f. Hymen
   g. Bartholin glands
3. The internal genital organs include:
   a. Vagina
   b. Uterus
   c. Fallopian tubes
   d. Ovaries
4. The female reproductive organs are under neurohormonal control
   a. The hypothalamus, anterior pituitary gland, and ovaries secrete hormones that operate by positive and negative feedback mechanisms
   b. The autonomic and spinal nerve pathways innervate the reproductive organs

C. Ectopic pregnancy

1. General information
   a. Ectopic pregnancy involves implantation of the fetus outside the uterine cavity
   b. Most ectopic pregnancies occur in the fallopian tubes, more commonly in the right tube than the left
   c. At least 75% of ectopic pregnancies are diagnosed in the first trimester and are symptomatic

      d. Fetal mortality is close to 100%; if diagnosis is delayed, maternal morbidity is high

2. Causes
   a. Tubal damage from pelvic inflammatory disease
   b. Congenital fallopian tube abnormalities
   c. Hormonal deficiencies
   d. Adhesions from previous abdominal surgery

3. Assessment findings (occur only after the fallopian tube ruptures)
   a. Sharp unilateral abdominal pain
   b. Syncope
   c. Referred shoulder pain
   d. Profuse vaginal bleeding

4. Diagnostic test findings
   a. Pelvic examination: pelvic mass and tenderness
   b. Culdocentesis: aspiration of nonclotted blood
   c. Ultrasonography: ectopic location of fetus
   d. Laparoscopy: nonruptured tubal pregnancy, if culdocentesis is not performed
   e. Laparotomy: diagnosis and opportunity for treatment
   f. Complete blood count (CBC): decreased hemoglobin (Hb) and hematocrit (HCT)

5. Patient care management goal: to control hemorrhage, replace blood loss, remove ectopic pregnancy, and provide support to the patient and family
   a. Type and crossmatch for possible blood transfusions to replace lost blood volume
   b. Prepare the patient and family for surgery
   c. Perform immediate laparoscopy to confirm diagnosis
   d. Consider hysterectomy for ruptured interstitial or cornual pregnancy; remove ovary if ovarian pregnancy
   e. Establish a large-bore I.V. line to gain access for adequate fluid replacement and possible blood administration
   f. Assess for shock; monitor for increased heart rate, decreased blood pressure, diaphoresis, and pallor
   g. Assess and document continuous ECG rhythm; vital signs; heart, lung, and bowel sounds; urine output; and any signs and symptoms indicating changes in these parameters
   h. Assess the patient's emotional state and coping mechanisms to evaluate the impact of losing the child
   i. Recognize that this is a crisis for the family
   j. Explain the diagnosis and implications to the patient and family to aid decision making about future pregnancies
   k. Refer the patient and family to community resources that can provide support, such as social services, counseling, and local support groups

D. Placenta previa
1. General information
   a. Placenta previa occurs when the placenta implants in the lower uterine segment
   b. Placenta previa may be total, partial, or low—according to the location of the implantation
   c. Because the lower uterine segment has less blood supply than the uterus, the placenta is forced to spread out over a wider area so it approaches or covers the cervical os
   d. The proximity of the placenta to the os increases the risk of infection from the vagina
   e. Postpartum hemorrhage may occur with the fundus firmly contracted
   f. Certain factors, such as age (35 or older), high parity, and a history of placenta previa, may increase a pregnant patient's risk
2. Cause: unknown
3. Assessment findings
   a. Painless uterine bleeding, especially in the third trimester
   b. Normal uterine tone
   c. Leopold's maneuver: the fetus in a breech, oblique, or transverse position
   d. Port wine amniotic fluid
4. Diagnostic test findings
   a. Ultrasound: location of placenta previa
   b. Vaginal examination: placenta inside cervical os; because of danger of bleeding, this examination should be done only if ultrasound is not available
   c. CBC: decreased Hb and HCT if bleeding is present
5. Patient care management goal: to identify and treat the condition promptly, to prevent hemorrhage, and to deliver a healthy, mature newborn
   a. Maintain bed rest and elevate the head of the bed
   b. Provide fluid administration, usually with lactated Ringer's solution, through a large-bore I.V. to maintain fluid balance
   c. Type and crossmatch 2 units of blood to hold in case of hemorrhage
   d. Consider cesarean delivery if the placenta previa is greater than 30% or if excessive bleeding occurs
   e. Maintain electronic monitoring of the mother and fetus to prevent complications
   f. Assess and document continuous ECG rhythm; vital signs; neurologic status; heart, lung, and bowel sounds; urine output; fetal and maternal monitoring; and any signs and symptoms indicating changes in these parameters
   g. Weigh saturated perineal pads to assess maternal blood loss
   h. Measure fundal height to assess for rising fundus, which may reveal concealed bleeding
   i. Allow no rectal or vaginal examinations, to minimize the danger of bleeding

    j.   Prepare the patient and family emotionally and physically for delivery

    k.   Observe for meconium in the amniotic fluid; may indicate fetal distress

    l.   Provide emotional support to the patient and family

E. Abruptio placentae
1. Introduction
   a. Abruptio placentae involves premature separation of the placenta from the uterine wall
   b. It begins when the small arteries in the uterine wall degenerate, rupture, and hemorrhage, causing a severe decrease in blood flow to the placenta. Distended by the pregnancy, the uterus cannot contract and compress the torn vessels effectively, and hemorrhage continues
   c. Abruptio placentae is classified as marginal, central, or complete
   d. In *marginal abruptio placentae,* bleeding between the fetal membranes and the uterine wall escapes vaginally
   e. In *central abruptio placentae,* bleeding is concealed between the uterine wall and the placenta
   f. *Complete abruptio placentae* is marked by sudden profuse vaginal bleeding
   g. Abruptio placentae may be so slight as to prevent diagnosis until after delivery, or so severe as to cause serious maternal complications and fetal death
2. Causes
   a. Increased intrauterine pressure from multiple pregnancy or hydramnios
   b. Maternal hypertension
   c. High maternal parity or age
   d. Excessive maternal alcohol use or cigarette smoking
   e. Abdominal trauma
3. Assessment findings
   a. Dark red vaginal bleeding; quantity depends on the degree of placental separation
   b. Abdominal tenderness
   c. Abdominal rigidity
   d. Increased abdominal girth
   e. Signs of hypovolemic shock
4. Diagnostic test findings
   a. Ultrasonography: may be normal
   b. Coagulation values: decreased fibrinogen and platelet levels
5. Patient care management goal: to identify and treat the condition promptly, to restore blood loss, and to prevent complications
   a. Assist with fetal delivery, which may include procedures such as amniotomy, oxytocin stimulation, or cesarean delivery, depending on the patient's clinical condition
   b. Maintain electronic monitoring of the mother and fetus to detect any signs of distress or abnormalities

c. Begin fluid administration—usually lactated Ringer's solution through a large-bore I.V.—to maintain fluid volume

d. Type and crossmatch 3 units of blood for transfusion if necessary

e. Administer oxygen at a flow rate based on institutional policy and the patient's clinical condition to increase fetal oxygenation

f. Assess for early signs of disseminated intravascular coagulation (DIC), the most serious complication, such as bruising, petechiae, and bleeding from the nose, gums, or I.V. sites

g. Assess and document continuous ECG rhythm; vital signs; neurologic status; heart, lung, and bowel sounds; urine output; fetal and maternal monitoring; and any signs and symptoms indicating changes in these parameters

h. Weigh saturated perineal pads to assess the mother's blood loss

i. Measure fundal height to detect a rising fundus, which may reveal concealed bleeding

j. Assess the patient's emotional state and coping mechanisms

k. Prepare the patient for surgery, if indicated

l. Administer medications, as ordered, for discomfort, anemia, or uterine atony, and document the patient's response

m. Help the family identify community resources that will provide support, such as social services, counseling, and local support groups, if the fetus is nonviable

F. Pregnancy-induced hypertension

1. Introduction

   a. Pregnancy-induced hypertension (PIH) is defined as consistent blood pressure readings of more than 140/90 mm Hg, or an increase over baseline of 30 mm Hg in systolic pressure or 15 mm Hg in diastolic pressure developing during an established pregnancy

   b. PIH typically develops after 20 weeks' gestation and resolves after the 10th postpartum day

   c. PIH is classified as preeclampsia or eclampsia

   d. A syndrome known as HELLP (hemolysis, elevated liver function, and low platelet count) has been associated with severe preeclampsia

   e. PIH is a leading cause of maternal mortality

   f. Risk factors associated with PIH include primigravidity, multiple fetuses, vascular disease, molar pregnancy, family history, and deficiencies in dietary protein and water-soluble vitamins

2. Causes: unknown

3. Assessment findings

   a. Hypertension

   b. Sudden excessive weight gain

   c. Generalized edema

   d. Headaches

   e. Hyperreflexia

   f. Seizures

   g. Blurred or double vision

    h. Fetal growth retardation

    i. Fetal distress

4. Diagnostic test findings

    a. Blood pressure: elevated above defined levels (definitive test)

    b. Urinalysis: proteinuria

    c. Serum liver function tests: elevated serum glutamic-oxaloacetic transaminase, serum glutamic-pyruvic transaminase, bilirubin

    d. Serum platelets: decreased

    e. Serum creatinine: increased

    f. Serum blood urea nitrogen: increased

5. Patient care management goal: to diagnose the condition promptly, reduce blood pressure, prevent complications, and deliver a healthy, mature newborn

    a. Maintain complete patient bed rest to minimize metabolic demands

    b. Provide electronic monitoring of the mother and fetus to detect any signs of distress or abnormalities

    c. Administer a high-protein, moderate-sodium diet to prevent a dietary imbalance if the patient is alert and not experiencing seizures

    d. Administer an anticonvulsant drug, such as magnesium sulfate ($MgSO_4$), the drug of choice. However, before administering $MgSO_4$, check reflexes (knee, ankle, and biceps); do not give if reflexes are absent, urine output is less than 100 ml in last 4 hours, or respirations are less than 12 per minute, to prevent potentially life-threatening adverse reactions. Have calcium gluconate available as an antidote

    e. Administer a sedative agent, such as diazepam or phenobarbital, to encourage bed rest

    f. Administer an antihypertensive agent such as hydralazine to reduce blood pressure, and document the patient's response

    g. Assess and document continuous ECG rhythm; vital signs; neurologic status; heart, lung, and bowel sounds; urine output; fetal and maternal monitoring; and any signs and symptoms that indicate changes in these parameters

    h. Institute safety precautions to minimize harm to the mother and fetus: maintain seizure precautions; have emergency equipment readily available; place the patient in a darkened, quiet room and install padded side rails

    i. If seizures occur, protect the patient and record the onset, precipitating factors, type of seizure, duration, and aftermath; reassess fetal status after every seizure

    j. Test urine for proteinuria every hour or as indicated

    k. Assess for signs of abruptio placentae (see item E above)

    l. Begin preparing for delivery

    m. Discuss family planning needs with the patient and family because future pregnancy may need to be delayed

    n. Encourage the patient to verbalize a need for follow-up care; ensure that the underlying cause of hypertension is unrelated to pregnancy

    o. Help the patient plan an acceptable means of birth control, with the understanding that the patient is not a candidate for oral contraceptives

Points to Remember

Reproductive emergencies create a crisis for the mother and family and may cause fetal death.

The patient's deep tendon reflexes should be checked before administering magnesium sulfate ($MgSO_4$).

No rectal or vaginal examinations should be performed on a patient with placenta previa.

DIC is one of the most serious complications in a patient with abruptio placentae.

Glossary

Amniotomy—artificial rupture of the fetal membranes

Atony—absence of muscle tone

Culdocentesis—use of an incision or needle puncture, through the vaginal wall, to remove intraperitoneal fluid

Laparoscopy—internal examination of the abdomen by inserting a small telescope through the anterior abdominal wall and filling the abdomen with carbon dioxide, allowing visualization of the abdominal organs

Leopold's maneuver—four palpation maneuvers of the mother's abdomen to evaluate fetal position

Disorders Affecting Multiple Systems

Learning Objectives

After studying this section, the reader should be able to:

- Describe the general principles of caring for a patient with a disorder affecting multiple systems.

- Identify possible causes for each type of disorder affecting multiple systems.

- Discuss common assessment and diagnostic test findings for the patient with specific disorders affecting multiple systems.

- Describe care management for the patient with a specific disorder affecting multiple systems.

XIX. Disorders Affecting Multiple Systems

A. Basic concepts

1. Various conditions have a profound impact on many body systems
2. The critical care and emergency nurse must anticipate this impact by integrating information and establishing patient care priorities
3. The critical care and emergency nurse must deal with critical situations with a precision and speed not usually required in other health care settings
4. Potential nursing diagnoses for the patient with a disorder affecting multiple body systems relate to the systems involved and include:
   a. Alteration in cardiac output
   b. Alteration in tissue perfusion
   c. Impaired gas exchange

B. Disseminated intravascular coagulation

1. Introduction
   a. Disseminated intravascular coagulation (DIC) disrupts normal coagulation, producing simultaneous clotting and bleeding
   b. DIC occurs as a secondary complication of another disease process
   c. Activation of the extrinsic or intrinsic coagulation pathway by the primary disease causes an abnormal acceleration of clotting
   d. Fibrinolysis results from the conversion of plasminogen to plasmin, a proteolytic enzyme
   e. Plasmin digests fibrinogen and fibrin and produces fibrin degradation products (FDPs)
   f. FDPs have an anticoagulant effect
   g. The processes of coagulation, anticoagulation, and fibrinolysis deplete clotting factors and predispose the patient to hemorrhage
   h. Most patients with DIC have had an episode of hypotension
2. Causes
   a. Trauma
   b. Burns
   c. Surgery
   d. Anaphylactic reactions
   e. Transfusion reactions
   f. Shock
   g. Fat or pulmonary embolism
   h. Prolonged extracorporeal circulation
   i. Transplant rejection
   j. Cirrhosis
   k. Sepsis
   l. Leukemia or other malignancy
   m. Obstetric emergencies such as abruptio placentae, amniotic fluid embolism, or unaborted dead fetus
3. Assessment findings
   a. Sudden onset of bleeding from trauma or surgical wounds
   b. Oozing from body orifices, mucosal surfaces, and venipuncture sites

      c. Hematuria

      d. Hematemesis

      e. Hemoptysis

      f. Guaiac-positive stool or gastric drainage

      g. Ecchymoses

      h. Petechiae or mottled skin

      i. Tachycardia, hypotension, and signs of shock

      j. Hypotension

      k. Irritability or confusion

4. Diagnostic test findings

      a. Chest X-ray: interstitial edema associated with lung microemboli

      b. ECG: ST segment changes indicating ischemia

      c. Arterial blood gas (ABG) measurements: acidosis

      d. Fibrinogen levels: decreased (fibrinogen is consumed by clot formation)

      e. Fibrin split products (FSPs): increased (produced by clot dissolution

      f. Prothrombin time (PT) and partial thromboplastin time (PTT): increased—caused by a depletion of coagulation factors

      g. Platelet count: decreased—caused by the removal of platelets from circulation to form clots

      h. Clotting factors V and VIII: reduced

      i. Peripheral blood smear: the presence of fragmented red blood cells (RBCs)—caused by the deposit of fibrin in the small blood vessels

5. Patient care management goal: to stop the bleeding by terminating the accelerated coagulation process

      a. Treat the underlying disease process

      b. Administer oxygen if hypoxia is present

      c. Administer continuous I.V. heparin. (This treatment may be controversial because of the increased risk of hemorrhaging, but heparin interferes with the clotting cascade at several sites and deactivates the fibrinolytic system, helping to minimize clot formation)

      d. Administer blood component transfusion, using fresh frozen plasma, cryoprecipitate, packed RBCs, and platelets to replace the clotting factors. Blood replacement should follow I.V. heparin, or the accelerated coagulation process will rapidly consume the blood products

      e. Prepare the patient for pulmonary artery catheter placement for monitoring fluid status and evaluating therapy

      f. Assess and document central venous pressure, pulmonary artery pressure (PAP), pulmonary artery wedge pressure (PAWP), cardiac output (CO), and systemic vascular resistance (SVR) as ordered

      g. Assess and document continuous ECG rhythm; vital signs; mental status; heart, lung, and bowel sounds; urine output; and any signs and symptoms indicating changes in these parameters

      h. Suction as necessary, taking care not to traumatize fragile tissue and trigger bleeding

      i. Before administering any other drugs, determine their compatibility or incompatibility with heparin

    j. Monitor results of coagulation studies and report any abnormal values

    k. Avoid giving I.M. injections to decrease risk of hematoma

    l. Offer the patient frequent oral care using nontraumatizing devices

    m. Institute protective measures to prevent skin damage such as lotion, pressure-relief devices, and position changes

    n. Provide a safe environment to prevent falls, tissue injury, and bruising

    o. Prevent transmission of infection by washing hands thoroughly and wearing gloves when contact with blood or body fluids is likely

    p. Teach the patient to recognize and report the signs and symptoms of coagulopathy if they recur or if chronic conditions such as leukemia exist

C. Shock: Cardiogenic

  1. Introduction

    a. Cardiogenic shock is a circulatory disturbance caused by inadequate cardiac pumping from severe left ventricular damage

    b. Cardiogenic shock, as a complication of myocardial infarction (MI), typically occurs when about 40% of the left ventricular wall is impaired

    c. The degree of impaired myocardial contractility is related to the size of the MI

    d. Two major changes in hemodynamic performance associated with cardiogenic shock include decreased CO and increased left ventricular end-diastolic pressure

    e. These changes initiate a cycle of decreased systemic perfusion, decreased coronary blood flow, increased myocardial ischemia, and reduced myocardial contractility

    f. Cardiogenic shock usually is fatal

  2. Causes

    a. MI

    b. Chronic progressive cardiomyopathy

    c. Ventricular septal rupture

    d. Papillary muscle rupture

    e. Ventricular aneurysm

  3. Assessment findings

    a. Systolic blood pressure less than 90 mm Hg or 30 mm Hg less than baseline values

    b. Oliguria, with urine output less than 20 ml/hr

    c. Rapid, thready pulse

    d. Cold, clammy skin

    e. Dyspnea

    f. Tachypnea

    g. Anxiety

    h. Confusion

    i. S_3 or S_4 heart sounds

    j. Crackles

4. Diagnostic test findings
   a. Cardiac index: less than 2.2 liters/min/m²
   b. PAWP: greater than 18 mm Hg
   c. Chest X-ray: cardiac enlargement and signs of left ventricular failure (pulmonary congestion)
   d. Echocardiogram: abnormalities of left ventricular wall motion and valve competency
   e. Serum chemistries: increased blood urea nitrogen (BUN), creatinine, and potassium
   f. Urinalysis: decreased specific gravity
   g. Urine creatinine clearance: decreased
   h. ABG measurements: decreased pH and bicarbonate (HCO_3^-)
5. Patient care management goal: to improve myocardial contractility, reduce myocardial work load, and decrease sodium and water retention
   a. Administer oxygen at a flow rate based on institutional policy and the patient's clinical condition to relieve ischemia; if gas exchange is inadequate, prepare the patient and the equipment for intubation
   b. Assess and document continuous ECG rhythm; vital signs; mental status; heart, lung, and bowel sounds; urine output; and any signs and symptoms that indicate changes in these parameters
   c. If a pulmonary artery catheter is in place, assess and document CVP, PAP, PAWP, CO, and SVR
   d. Place the patient in a supine position with legs slightly elevated, to promote blood flow to the brain
   e. Administer inotropic agents, as ordered, to improve myocardial contractility and CO
   f. Administer vasopressors, as ordered, to improve blood pressure
   g. Monitor intra-aortic balloon pump, if inserted, to improve coronary artery perfusion and reduce afterload
   h. Administer diuretics, as ordered, to reduce preload and improve CO
   i. Administer vasodilators, as ordered, to reduce afterload
   j. Prepare for emergency percutaneous transluminal coronary angioplasty (PTCA) to improve blood flow through stenotic coronary arteries
   k. Recognize that emergency coronary artery bypass graft surgery may be indicated to reperfuse ischemic areas; alternately, a left ventricular assist device or heart transplantation may be indicated

D. Shock: Anaphylactic
1. Introduction
   a. Anaphylactic shock is a hypersensitivity reaction to an allergen, marked by extreme respiratory distress
   b. The reaction occurs in a person who has previously been exposed to the antigen and who has built up antibodies against it
   c. Anaphylactic shock is a type of vasogenic shock
   d. Untreated, it can lead to respiratory arrest and tissue hypoxia

2. Causes
   a. Drugs, most commonly penicillin
   b. Anesthetic agents
   c. Blood transfusions
   d. Insect stings or bites
3. Assessment findings
   a. Dyspnea
   b. Air hunger
   c. Complete airway obstruction
   d. Systolic blood pressure less than 90 mm Hg or 30 mm Hg less than baseline value
   e. Palpitations
   f. Nausea and vomiting
   g. Urticaria
   h. Swelling of eyes, lips, tongue, hands, feet, and genitalia
4. Diagnostic test findings
   a. Diagnosis is based on presenting signs and symptoms
   b. IgE serum levels: elevated (may confirm allergic reaction as origin)
5. Patient care management goal: to maintain a patent airway and to counteract the effects of anaphylaxis
   a. Prepare the patient and the equipment for intubation if gas exchange is inadequate.
   b. Administer epinephrine to dilate bronchioles, inhibit and counteract histamine response, and increase myocardial contractility
   c. Administer oxygen at a flow rate based on institutional policy and the patient's clinical condition to relieve hypoxia
   d. Assess and document continuous ECG rhythm; vital signs; mental status; heart, lung, and bowel sounds; urine output; and any signs and symptoms that indicate changes in these parameters
   e. If a pulmonary artery catheter is in place, assess and document CVP, PAP, PAWP, CO, and SVR as ordered
   f. Begin fluid therapy with colloids and crystalloids to restore adequate vascular volume
   g. Consider vasopressors if fluids are not successful
   h. Provide antihistamines to relieve itching
   i. Consider bronchodilators to relieve bronchospasm
   j. Place the patient in a supine position with legs slightly elevated to promote blood flow to the brain
   k. Teach the patient to identify and avoid potential causative antigens
   l. Encourage the patient to wear a Medic Alert bracelet and to notify medical personnel of allergy
   m. Teach the family how to use an emergency anaphylaxis kit at home and how to activate the emergency medical system

E. Shock: Septic

1. Introduction
   a. Septic shock is a life-threatening disorder caused by a bacterium, a virus, or a fungus in the bloodstream and leading to impaired cellular functioning and altered hemodynamic status
   b. Septic shock is a type of vasogenic shock
   c. Septic shock is the uncontrolled progression on a continuum that begins with bacteremia and leads to septicemia and septic shock
   d. It most commonly occurs when the body's defense against infection is impaired or normal protective barriers are disrupted
   e. Patients at risk include those who have recently undergone traumatic injuries, surgery, or invasive procedures, and those who are malnourished, immunocompromised, or debilitated
   f. Gram-negative organisms are implicated in 70% of cases. (For this reason, this coverage focuses on management of gram-negative shock)
   g. The urinary tract is involved in about 50% of gram-negative infections
   h. Nosocomial infections are the most common cause of septic shock
   i. Broad-spectrum antibiotics are typically started after cultures are obtained but before sensitivity reports are available
   j. Septic shock is divided into two stages: early and late
   k. In *early sepsis,* beta stimulation leads to increased CO but also to decreased cardiac filling pressure and SVR because of vasodilation
   l. In *late sepsis,* CO decreases and filling pressure increases as the heart fails; SVR is increased because of the vasoconstriction produced by the release of catecholamines and prostaglandins
2. Causes
   a. Infection
   b. Immunosuppressant therapy
3. Assessment findings
   a. Systolic blood pressure less than 90 mm Hg or 30 mm Hg less than baseline
   b. Tachycardia
   c. Cool, clammy skin
   d. Pallor
   e. Oliguria
4. Diagnostic test findings
   a. ABG measurements: respiratory alkalosis progressing to respiratory acidosis
   b. Serum chemistries: increased BUN, creatinine, lactate, and potassium; decreased HCO_3^-
   c. Complete blood count (CBC): increased leukocytes and neutrophils
   d. Blood cultures: positive for causative agent
   e. SVR: decreased
   f. PT and PTT: increased

5. Patient care management goal: to treat the causative organism, reverse vasodilation, and maintain tissue perfusion
   a. Administer oxygen at a flow rate based on institutional policy and the patient's clinical condition to relieve hypoxia
   b. Assess and document continuous ECG rhythm; vital signs; mental status; heart, lung, and bowel sounds; urine output; and any signs and symptoms indicating changes in these parameters
   c. If a pulmonary artery catheter is in place, assess and document CVP, PAP, PAWP, CO, and SVR as ordered
   d. Administer antibiotics as ordered to combat infection, and document the patient's response
   e. Place the patient in a supine position with legs slightly elevated to aid venous return
   f. If gas exchange is inadequate, prepare the patient and equipment for intubation
   g. Administer inotropic agents to augment contractility and CO
   h. Administer vasopressors to reverse vasodilation
   i. Consider administering steroids to decrease inflammatory response
   j. Use antipyretics and cooling blankets to maintain the patient's body temperature within an acceptable range, thus decreasing metabolic demands
   k. Consider nutritional support to maintain adequate nutrition, if the patient's oral intake is insufficient
   l. Consider administering naloxone hydrochloride to help correct vasodilation

F. **Shock: Hypovolemic**
   1. Introduction
      a. Hypovolemic shock reduces CO and causes inadequate tissue perfusion from a loss of circulating blood volume
      b. Surgical patients are at high risk because of blood loss intraoperatively and trauma from the manipulation of body tissues (see Section XIV, item G, "Fluid volume disturbances," for more information)
   2. Causes
      a. Hemorrhage
      b. Burns
      c. Dehydration
      d. Trauma
   3. Assessment findings
      a. Systolic blood pressure less than 90 mm Hg or 30 mm Hg less than baseline values
      b. Tachycardia
      c. Decreased PAWP
      d. Cool, clammy skin
      e. Pallor

      f. Oliguria

      g. Extreme thirst

      h. Irritability

  4. Diagnostic test findings

      a. ABG measurements: respiratory alkalosis progressing to respiratory acidosis

      b. Serum chemistries: increased BUN, creatinine, lactate, and potassium; decreased HCO_3^-

      c. CBC: increased hematocrit (HCT)

  5. Patient care management goal: to restore the circulating blood volume

      a. Assess and document continuous ECG rhythm; vital signs; mental status; heart, lung, and bowel sounds; urine output; and any signs and symptoms indicating changes in these parameters

      b. Administer fluids (LR or NS) to correct fluid deficit

      c. If a pulmonary artery catheter is in place, assess the patient's fluid volume and document CVP, PAP, PAWP, CO, and SVR as ordered

      d. Weigh the patient daily at the same time and on the same scale; note changes and any trends

      e. Administer oxygen at a flow rate based on institutional policy and the patient's clinical condition to relieve ischemia

      f. Place the patient in a supine position with legs slightly elevated to promote blood flow to the brain

      g. If gas exchange is inadequate, prepare the patient and equipment for intubation

G. Shock: Neurogenic

  1. Introduction

      a. Neurogenic shock causes loss of overall vasomotor tone, leading to massive vasodilation and relative hypovolemia

      b. The disorder is a form of distributive shock

  2. Causes

      a. Deep general or spinal anesthesia

      b. Brain or spinal cord damage

      c. Prolonged medullary ischemia

      d. Overdose of barbiturates or adrenergic and ganglionic blocking agents

  3. Assessment findings

      a. Warm, dry, possibly flushed skin

      b. Systolic blood pressure less than 90 mm Hg or 30 mm Hg less than baseline values

      c. Full, regular pulse

      d. Profound bradycardia

      e. Poikilothermy (body temperature that varies with environmental temperature)

  4. Diagnostic test findings

      a. SVR: decreased

      b. ABG measurements: decreased pH and HCO_3^-

5. Patient care management goal: to improve vasomotor tone, reverse vasodilation, and maintain tissue perfusion
   a. Assess and document continuous ECG rhythm; vital signs; mental status; heart, lung, and bowel sounds; urine output; and any signs and symptoms indicating changes in these parameters
   b. If a pulmonary artery catheter is in place, assess the patient's fluid volume and document CVP, PAP, PAWP, CO, and SVR as ordered
   c. Administer oxygen at a flow rate based on institutional policy and the patient's clinical condition to relieve ischemia
   d. Place the patient in a supine position with legs slightly elevated to aid venous return, unless cerebral edema is suspected
   e. Perform neurologic checks (using the Glasgow Coma Scale), including pupillary response, and report changes from baseline
   f. Administer vasopressors to reverse vasodilation
   g. Observe for a spontaneous resolution of neurogenic shock if induced by anesthesia

H. Burns

1. Introduction
   a. Burns refer to any damage to the skin or body tissue caused by thermal, electrical, chemical, or radiation injury
   b. Damage interferes with normal skin functions, compromises protection against infection, causes loss of body fluids, alters control of body temperature, interferes with vitamin D activation, alters sensory and excretory functions, and diminishes body image
   c. The extent and depth of injury relates to the intensity and duration of exposure to the source of injury
   d. Regardless of etiology, the basic principles of burn care remain the same
   e. Skin damage from burns is commonly defined in terms of the skin layers involved, either partial thickness or full thickness
   f. *Partial-thickness burns* can be further classified as superficial (or first degree) and deep partial (or second degree)
   g. *Full-thickness* (or *third-degree*) *burns* destroy all skin layers and may damage nerves, muscles, bones, and blood vessels
   h. The extent of burns in adults can be estimated quickly by using the Rule of Nines
   i. Estimating the extent of burns in children involves using a chart (known as the Lund and Browder chart) that considers changes in the size of body parts with growth
   j. Three phases of burn care include the emergent, the acute, and the rehabilitation phases
   k. The *emergent* phase begins immediately after the injury as the body reacts with an inflammatory response and a large shift of extracellular fluid to the damaged tissues; this phase usually lasts 2 to 4 days

(Text continues on page 194.)

RULE OF NINES

This method for estimating the extent of an adult patient's burns divides body surface area into percentages that, when totaled, equal 100%. To use this method, mentally transfer the patient's burns to the body chart shown here, then add up the corresponding percentages for each burned body section. The total, a rough estimate of the extent of the patient's burns, enters into the formula to determine his initial fluid replacement needs.

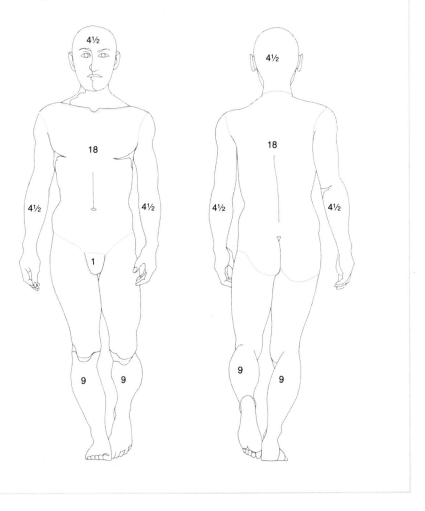

THE LUND AND BROWDER CHART

The Rule of Nines is a quick way to roughly estimate the percentage of your patient's body surface that's been burned. But it can't be used for infants and children because their body section percentages differ from those of adults.

To determine the extent of an infant's or child's burns, use the Lund and Browder chart shown here. This chart takes proportional age-size differences into account.

RELATIVE PERCENTAGES OF AREAS AFFECTED BY GROWTH						
	At birth	1 year	5 years	10 years	15 years	Adult
A: Half of head	9½%	8½%	6½%	5½%	4½%	3½%
B: Half of thigh	2¾%	3¼%	4%	4¼%	4½%	4¾%
C: Half of leg	2½%	2½%	2¾%	3%	3¼%	3½%

    l. The *acute* phase occurs as the body attempts to heal the wound and prevent infection; this phase begins at the end of the emergent phase and lasts until the injury is healed (either spontaneously or with grafting)

    m. The *rehabilitation* phase occurs as the patient attempts to return to optimal level of function

    n. Education on burn prevention is vital because most burns are caused by carelessness, ignorance, or curiosity

2. Assessment findings: partial-thickness

    a. Superficial burn: pink or red skin, small blisters, pain eased by cooling, skin blanching on pressure

    b. Deep partial burn: large blisters; edema; wet, weeping, and shiny surface; pain and sensitivity to cold air

3. Assessment findings: full-thickness

    a. Deep-red, black, or white appearance

    b. Edema

    c. Exposed subcutaneous fat layer

    d. Little or no pain

    e. Signs and symptoms of shock

4. Diagnostic test findings

    a. ABG measurements: decreased partial pressures of oxygen in arterial blood (PaO_2) and increased or decreased partial pressures of carbon dioxide in arterial blood ($PaCO_2$)

    b. Culture and sensitivity tests: infection (burn sepsis is defined as 10^5 microorganisms/gram burn tissue)

    c. Carboxyhemoglobin level: positive with smoke inhalation

    d. Serum chemistries: increased potassium and decreased sodium and total protein

    e. CBC: increased HCT initially; decreased Hb

    f. Creatine phosphokinase levels: elevated with electrical burns, with degree of elevation indicating amount of muscle injury

5. Patient care management is determined by the extent of injury and phase of care; general goals of therapy include:

    a. Assess and document continuous ECG rhythm; vital signs; mental status; heart, lung, and bowel sounds; urine output; and any signs and symptoms indicating changes in these parameters

    b. If a pulmonary artery catheter is in place, assess and document CVP, PAP, PAWP, CO, and SVR as ordered

    c. Maintain a patent airway by proper positioning, removal of secretions, and maintenance of artificial airway, if present

    d. Observe for blistering of lips, singed nasal hairs, increased hoarseness, and soot in sputum indicating injury to the respiratory tract

    e. Administer small, frequent I.V. doses of narcotics for pain relief; avoid I.M. injections for pain control until the patient is hemodynamically stable and adequate tissue perfusion is achieved

    f. Estimate the percentage of body surface area involved using the Rule of Nines or the Lund and Browder chart

g. Begin fluid and electrolyte replacement based on institutional protocol and the patient's needs

h. Administer tetanus toxoid to combat anaerobic infections

i. Elevate the head of the bed and the burned patient's extremities to prevent edema

j. Assess wounds for local signs of infection such as drainage, swelling, redness, or poor graft take

k. Keep the patient warm with blankets, heat lamps, and heat shields to maintain body temperature

l. Keep the patient on nothing-by-mouth status and provide low wall suction to nasogastric tube to relieve nausea and vomiting until bowel sounds return

m. Evaluate the patient's response to wound treatments such as cleaning, debridement, whirlpool, antibacterial therapy, dressing changes, or skin grafting

n. Assess the patient's nutritional intake, providing high-calorie nutritional support to ensure that metabolic needs are met

o. Provide patient education to ensure that the patient and family can recognize the importance of support groups, use exercises and splints correctly, list food high in protein and calories important in wound healing, and understand the need for follow-up care

Points to Remember

In DIC, the processes of coagulation, anticoagulation, and fibrinolysis deplete clotting factors and cause hemorrhage.

Regardless of the type of shock, inadequate oxygen delivery to the tissues is the primary hemodynamic mechanism.

An anaphylactic reaction occurs in a person who has had previous exposure to an antigen and has developed antibodies to it.

Nosocomial infections are the most common cause of septic shock.

Most burn injuries are caused by carelessness, ignorance, or curiosity, so education about prevention is vital.

Glossary

Antigen—substance that causes an antibody

Fibrinolysis—destruction of fibrin by enzymatic digestion of cells

Vasogenic shock—type of shock causing profound vasodilation from an increase in total vascular capacity

Trauma

Learning Objectives

After studying this section, the reader should be able to:

- Describe the general principles of trauma.

- Identify possible causes for each type of trauma.

- Discuss common assessment and diagnostic test findings for the patient with a specific traumatic injury.

- Describe care management for the patient with a specific traumatic injury.

XX. Trauma

A. Basic concepts

1. Trauma is injury occurring from force; it may be accidental, self-inflicted, or an act of violence that affects multiple systems and requires immediate and specialized interventions to prevent loss of limb or life
2. Trauma victims commonly have injury to more than one body system
3. It is the leading cause of death for persons age 1 to 44
4. The emergence of trauma care centers with capabilities of sophisticated emergency interventions has significantly decreased mortality and morbidity from traumatic injury
5. Common causes of trauma
   a. Motor vehicle accidents, including auto, motorcycle, and pedestrian
   b. Gunshot wounds
   c. Stab wounds with knives or other sharp objects
   d. Falls
   e. Sports-related injuries
6. Trauma is classified as blunt or penetrating
   a. *Blunt trauma* is associated with accidents, such as motor vehicle accidents or falls
   b. *Penetrating trauma* is associated with injuries, such as stab wounds, gunshot wounds, or impalement
7. Risk factors commonly associated with trauma
   a. Alcohol and drug use
   b. Sex: Males have twice the risk of fatal injury as females
   c. Age: Persons age 15 to 24 have the highest number of traumatic injuries; elderly people have the highest number of fatal injuries
8. Assessment findings depend on the systems that are injured, but the *cardinal rules in multiple trauma* should be applied

---

CARDINAL RULES IN MULTIPLE TRAUMA

- All patients with head and facial trauma have a cervical spine injury.
- All patients with an altered level of consciousness have a head injury.
- All young, healthy patients lacking a palpable radial pulse are in shock.
- Hypotension, tachycardia, and pallor indicate bleeding into the chest, abdomen, or pelvis if no obvious external injuries are present.
- All patients with chest trauma are presumed critical.
- All patients with distended neck veins have pericardial tamponade or tension pneumothorax.
- Penetrating wounds at or below the nipple line involve the chest and abdomen.
- Systolic blood pressure is estimated to be: Palpable radial pulse = 80 to 100 mm Hg Palpable femoral pulse = 70 mm Hg.

Reprinted with permission from N. Holloway, *Nursing the Critically Ill Adult*, 3rd ed. Menlo Park, Calif.: Addison-Wesley Publishing Co., 1988.

9. Potential nursing diagnoses for the patient suffering trauma include:
   a. Ineffective airway clearance
   b. Ineffective breathing pattern
   c. Impaired gas exchange
   d. Alteration in cardiac output: decreased
   e. Alteration in tissue perfusion
   f. Fluid volume deficit
   g. Impaired physical mobility
   h. Alteration in comfort: pain

B. Head trauma
1. Introduction
   a. Head trauma occurs following blunt or penetrating injuries to the cranial or cerebral structures; it includes skull fractures and damage to brain tissue
   b. Acceleration head injury is caused by a moving object striking the head
   c. Deceleration head injury is caused by the head striking a stationary object
   d. Types of head injuries include concussion, contusion, cranial fractures, epidural or subdural hematoma, subarachnoid hemorrhage, and herniation
   e. Abnormal flexion (decorticate positioning) is seen in head-injury patients with hemispheric dysfunction
   f. Abnormal extension (decerebrate positioning) is seen in head-injury patients with brain stem injury
2. Assessment findings: concussion
   a. Nausea
   b. Vomiting
   c. Amnesia
   d. Dizziness
   e. Irritability
   f. Sluggishness
   g. Disorientation or confusion
   h. Visual disturbances
3. Assessment findings: contusion
   a. Altered level of consciousness (LOC)
   b. Nausea
   c. Vomiting
   d. Visual disturbances
   e. Weakness
   f. Ataxia
   g. Speech problems
   h. Hemiparesis
   i. Seizures

4. Assessment findings: cranial fractures (findings depend on type and site of fracture)
   a. Altered LOC
   b. Headache
   c. Swelling
   d. Hematoma
   e. Pain
   f. Nausea
   g. Vomiting
   h. Diaphoresis
   i. Rhinorrhea or otorrhea
   j. Periorbital ecchymosis or other evidence of bleeding
5. Assessment findings: epidural hematoma (rapid deterioration)
   a. Altered LOC
   b. Headache
   c. Hemiparesis
   d. Dilated pupil on side of injury
   e. Bradycardia
   f. Hypertension
6. Assessment findings: subdural hematoma (similar to stroke, tumor, or senility)
   a. Headache
   b. Fever
   c. Unilateral pupil dilation
   d. Papilledema
   e. Hemiparesis or plegia
7. Assessment findings: subarachnoid hemorrhage
   a. Piercing headache
   b. Nuchal rigidity
   c. Photophobia
   d. Nausea
   e. Vomiting
   f. Delirium
   g. Altered LOC
   h. Syncope
   i. Irritability
   j. Coma
   k. Respiratory distress
   l. Dilated pupils
   m. Papilledema
   n. Retinal hemorrhage
   o. Focal motor signs such as twitching
   p. Seizures
8. Assessment findings: herniation
   a. Altered LOC
   b. Hemiparesis

    c. Respiratory distress

    d. Positive Babinski reflex

9. Diagnostic test findings

    a. X-rays: reveal spinal, cervical, or skull fracture

    b. Computed tomography (CT) scan: identifies type, location, and extent of injury

    c. Cerebral angiography: locates area of injury

    d. Electroencephalogram: locates area of irritability; shows absence of brain activity; determines presence of brain death

10. Patient care management goal: to control intracranial pressure (ICP) and to prevent secondary injury and complications

    a. Monitor ICP to maintain cerebral perfusion pressure (CPP) at 60 to 80 mm Hg

    b. Treat increased ICP by elevating the head of bed, loosening any tight garments around the neck that might impede venous return, and checking for other causes of increased ICP such as abdominal or bladder distention or anxiety

    c. Maintain normotensive blood pressure because both hypotension and hypertension can increase cerebral edema

    d. Administer I.V. fluids (dextrose 5% in water [D_5W] with normal saline solution; plain D_5W can cause cerebral edema)

    e. Maintain normal body temperature to prevent hyperthermia, which increases metabolic demand

    f. Administer anticonvulsive medications to prevent seizures (may be given prophylactically)

    g. Administer diuretics and glucocorticoids to decrease cerebral edema and ICP

    h. Administer paralyzing agents such as pancuronium bromide to reduce skeletal muscle response and lower the risk of intracranial hypertension; the patient must be intubated and mechanically ventilated

    i. Administer barbiturates to induce coma, which reduces the cerebral metabolic rate and decreases intracranial hypertension; the patient must be intubated and mechanically ventilated

    j. Avoid the use of narcotics because they mask changes in LOC and impair neurologic assessment

    k. Monitor arterial blood gas (ABG) measurements to maintain levels of partial pressures of carbon dioxide in arterial blood at less than 35 mm Hg because higher levels increase ICP

    l. Avoid coughing exercises, which increase ICP

    m. Test any drainage from the nose or ears for glucose (will test positive if drainage is cerebrospinal fluid [CSF])

    n. Assess neurologic status and LOC frequently to detect subtle changes

    o. Prepare the patient for surgical intervention, if necessary, to evacuate hematoma, elevate depressed skull fracture, remove any foreign objects, and repair tears or aneurysm

    p. Encourage the patient to report any aura that precedes seizure activity

    q. Encourage the patient's participation in self-care and rehabilitation

C. Spinal cord injury
1. Introduction
    a. Spinal cord injury (SCI) is trauma to the spinal cord caused by hemorrhage, concussion, contusion, laceration, or diminished blood supply
    b. SCI may be referred to by type and etiology as complete or incomplete, or by level of injury
    c. Because of the greater range of mobility in the vertebral column in certain areas, the vertebrae most commonly injured include the 5th, 6th, and 7th cervical; the 12th thoracic; and the 1st lumbar
    d. SCI severity depends on the spinal area injured
    e. Prompt and proper handling of the patient at the accident scene can reduce further damage and preserve remaining neurologic function
    f. Of the 15,000 to 20,000 patients who sustain SCI each year, about 50% are rendered quadriplegic and the other 50% are paraplegic
    g. Patients with injury at or above T6 often experience autonomic dysreflexia (AD), a life-threatening response to a stimulus by the autonomic nervous system, most commonly resulting from a stimulus to the bladder. Classic signs and symptoms include headache, hypertension, cutaneous vasodilation, and diaphoresis above the injured spinal cord area
2. Assessment findings: depend on location and type of cord injury
    a. Neck or back pain
    b. Vertebral tenderness or deformity
    c. Extremity numbness or tingling
    d. Muscle weakness or paralysis
    e. Asymmetrical reflexes or absence of reflexes
    f. Bowel and bladder incontinence
    g. Hypotension
    h. Bradycardia
    i. Respiratory insufficiency
3. Diagnostic test findings
    a. Spinal X-ray: change in vertebral positioning and cord impingement
    b. CT scan: change in vertebral positioning and cord impingement
    c. Myelography: herniated intervertebral discs or blocked CSF flow
    d. Evoked potential studies and electromyography: area of spinal cord lesion
4. Patient care management goal: to immobilize the patient, restore normal position, stabilize the vertebral column, and prevent complications
    a. Stabilize the patient's spine to prevent further damage
    b. Use traction such as Harrington or Lanque for thoracolumbar injury immobilization
    c. Consider special devices for immobilization such as plaster jacket, Jewett nail, or Weiss spring
    d. Aid immobilization with bed frame devices with or without traction such as Stryker frame or kinetic beds with halo traction
    e. Anticipate surgery for spinal fracture or cord compression

GUIDE TO MOTOR AND SENSORY IMPAIRMENT IN SPINAL CORD INJURY

SPINAL AREA AFFECTED	TYPE OF MOTOR LOSS	AREA OF SENSORY LOSS (PAIN, TEMPERATURE, TOUCH, AND PRESSURE)
C1 to C4	• Diaphragm paresis • Intercostal paralysis • Flaccid total paralysis in skeletal muscles below neck	• Neck and below
C5 to C8	• Intercostal paralysis • Paralysis below shoulders and upper arms	• Arms and hands, chest, abdomen, and legs
T1 to T6	• Paralysis below midchest	• Below midchest
T7 to T12	• Paralysis below waist	• Below waist
L1 to L3	• Paralysis in most leg muscles and in pelvis	• Lower abdomen and legs
L4 to L5	• Paralysis in lower legs, ankles, feet	• Parts of lower legs and feet
S1 to S5	• Ataxic paralysis of the bladder and rectum • Paralysis of feet and ankles	• Posterior inner thigh, lateral foot, perineum

    f. Maintain patent airway for adequate oxygenation

    g. Consider using kinetic beds to help prevent complications of bed rest and to promote peristalsis and postural drainage

    h. Decrease severe pain with analgesics or narcotics

    i. Administer anti-inflammatory agents, such as dexamethasone, to decrease muscle pain

    j. Control muscle spasms with the use of muscle relaxants such as baclofen

    k. Assess the patient for signs and symptoms of ascending cord edema, including decreased sensory and motor loss greater than previously documented, change in respiratory pattern, or difficulty swallowing

    l. Evaluate for signs of AD; place the patient in a sitting position, correct the offending stimulus, and notify the doctor

    m. Minimize complications of bed rest: turn the patient frequently, perform active and passive range-of-motion exercises, apply antiembolism stockings, maintain adequate hydration, and use a pressure-relief mattress or therapeutic bed. Note: *Do not* turn the patient before the spinal cord has been stabilized

    n. Support the patient's psychosocial needs related to sexuality, self-esteem, and altered body image; help the patient and family cope, accept the changes, and plan for the future

    o. Begin bowel and bladder retraining program, as indicated, to achieve regularly predicted elimination and prevent bladder infection

  p. Direct the patient and family to community resources, such as social services, counseling, spinal cord associations, local support groups, and visiting nurses

  q. Have the patient and family demonstrate the use of assistive devices and perform exercises that promote maximum functioning

  r. Involve the patient and family in decisions regarding care and referral to rehabilitation centers

D. Chest trauma

1. Introduction

  a. Chest trauma occurs following a blunt or penetrating injury to the chest, which may involve damage to the bony structures of the thorax, the heart, or lungs

  b. Chest injuries are the second leading cause of death for trauma victims

  c. Both blunt and penetrating injuries can produce pneumothorax

  d. Penetrating objects should be removed by the doctor only after bleeding is controlled, because they can have a sealing effect and their removal can produce uncontrollable bleeding or pneumothorax

  e. Types of chest injuries include rib fractures (most commonly ribs 5 to 9), flail chest, myocardial or pulmonary contusion, cardiac tamponade, open pneumothorax, and hemothorax

2. Assessment findings

  a. Shortness of breath

  b. Chest pain, especially with respirations

  c. Tachypnea, nasal flaring, and other signs of ventilatory distress

  d. Paradoxical chest wall movement (with flail chest)

  e. Hemoptysis

  f. Diminished breath sounds

  g. Tracheal deviation with tension pneumothorax

  h. Subcutaneous crepitations

3. Diagnostic test findings

  a. Chest X-ray: fractures and air or fluid in the pleural space

  b. ABG measurements: acid-base imbalances and presence of hypoxemia

  c. ECG: dysrhythmias (a common complication of chest trauma)

  d. Complete blood count (CBC): decreased hemoglobin (Hb) and hematocrit (HCT)

4. Patient care management goal: to prevent respiratory compromise and complications from the injury

  a. Maintain patent airway

  b. Assess and document continuous ECG rhythm; vital signs; mental status; heart, lung, and bowel sounds; urine output; and any signs and symptoms that indicate changes in these parameters

  c. Replace lost blood with whole blood or packed cells

  d. Prepare the patient for chest tube insertion to remove accumulated fluid or air from the chest and allow reexpansion of the lung

  e. Prepare the patient for pulmonary artery catheter placement to monitor fluid status and evaluate therapy

     f. Assess and document central venous pressure, pulmonary artery pressure, pulmonary arterial wedge pressure, pulmonary vascular resistance, and systemic vascular resistance

     g. Prepare the patient for surgical intervention to stabilize flail chest or to evacuate massive hemothorax or tamponade

     h. Manage the patient's pain with nonnarcotics or intercostal nerve block so that respiration is not depressed

     i. Maintain patency and proper functioning of chest tube drainage system to ensure evacuation of drainage and air

     j. Monitor chest tube drainage for amount and color and document

     k. Provide chest tube dressing care according to institutional policy to prevent infection and promote healing

     l. Teach the patient to use breathing techniques to promote lung expansion and healing

E. Abdominal trauma

  1. Introduction

     a. Abdominal trauma occurs following a blunt or penetrating injury to the abdomen, which may cause injury to internal organs

     b. Solid organs such as the spleen, pancreas, kidneys, and uterus are typically injured by penetrating trauma

     c. Hollow organs, such as the stomach, bladder, and intestines, are typically injured by blunt trauma

     d. More than 50% of the patients with blunt trauma to the abdomen also have injury to the head, chest, or extremities

     e. Abdominal trauma commonly causes massive blood loss and shock

     f. Injury to retroperitoneal structures such as the pancreas and duodenum may cause blood loss of up to 4 liters, which may not be detected immediately

     g. The spleen is one of the most frequently injured organs, which may cause massive hemorrhage

     h. Injury to the abdominal aorta, inferior vena cava, or hepatic vessels may cause rapid, massive bleeding

  2. Assessment findings: may vary considerably; absence of signs and symptoms does not exclude major injury

     a. Abdominal pain, ranging from mild to severe

     b. Respiratory distress from abdominal distention

     c. Signs of hypovolemia such as decreased blood pressure, tachycardia, and pallor

     d. Wounds

     e. Abrasions

     f. Bruising on the abdomen

     g. Absent or decreased bowel sounds

     h. Decreased LOC

3. Diagnostic test findings
   a. X-rays: fractures, free air, fluid, or foreign objects
   b. CT scan: intraperitoneal and retroperitoneal bleeding
   c. CBC: decreased Hb and HCT
   d. White blood cell count: increased, indicating infection
   e. Serum glucose: elevated because of catecholamine release
   f. Serum amylase: elevated with injury to the pancreas and small bowel
   g. Liver enzymes (serum glutamic-oxaloacetic transaminase, serum glutamic-pyruvic transaminase, and lactate dehydrogenase): elevated, reflecting hepatic injury from trauma or ischemia
   h. Peritoneal lavage: intra-abdominal bleeding
4. Patient care management goal: to correct volume deficit and prevent complications of shock and infection
   a. Administer immediate fluid resuscitation with warmed saline or lactated Ringer's solution (may require use of pressure bags or infusion pumps to speed replacement)
   b. Replace lost blood with fresh whole blood; autotransfusion is avoided because of the risk of contamination
   c. Apply medical antishock trousers (MAST suit) to elevate blood pressure in cases of severe trauma
   d. Evaluate wound for signs of evisceration; if present, cover with wet saline and do not attempt to replace tissue
   e. Insert nasogastric tube to decompress stomach and remove gastric contents
   f. Insert urinary catheter to monitor renal function and aid in assessing genitourinary injury
   g. Administer broad-spectrum antibiotics prophylactically because of high probability of infection
   h. Administer nonnarcotic analgesics for pain management because narcotics decrease respiratory effort and alter sensorium
   i. Administer parenteral nutrition if GI function is impaired; initiate promptly to meet the patient's metabolic needs
   j. Prepare the patient for surgical intervention as indicated for wounds invading the peritoneum, GI hemorrhage, free air in abdomen, evisceration, massive hematuria, positive diagnostic peritoneal lavage
   k. Teach the patient to identify the signs and symptoms of possible bowel obstruction or infection that require medical attention

F. Limb trauma
   1. Introduction
      a. Limb trauma occurs following a blunt or penetrating injury to the upper or lower extremities
      b. Limb trauma occurs in all age-groups and is a major source of disability
      c. Most common types of limb trauma are strains, sprains, and fractures
      d. Strains are stretch injuries that occur to the muscle at the tendon site

    e. Sprains are ligament injuries that occur from a force greater than that which causes a strain

    f. Strains and sprains are caused by any kind of movement or a wrenching force

    g. Fractures are a disruption or break in a bone

    h. Fractures commonly are caused by a force or penetrating object that is sufficient to crack or break the bone

    i. Prompt management is essential to prevent additional damage or loss of the limb

2. Assessment findings: strains and sprains

    a. Pain

    b. Swelling

    c. Point tenderness

    d. Discoloration

    e. Muscle spasm

    f. Brief loss of function

3. Assessment findings: fractures

    a. Pain

    b. Swelling

    c. Tenderness

    d. Discoloration

    e. Muscle spasm

    f. Loss of movement

    g. Deformity or angulation of limb

    h. Protrusion of bone fragments (compound fracture)

4. Diagnostic test findings: limb X-ray identifies the location and type of fracture (no specific tests for strains or sprains)

5. Patient care management goal: to immobilize the affected area to allow healing and prevent further injury

    a. Immobilize the strain or sprain with a compression bandage

    b. Immobilize the limb above and below the fracture site, using a splint, cast, surgical pins, sling, or traction

    c. Apply a cold pack for 24 to 48 hours to decrease swelling

    d. Assess limb color, temperature, capillary refill, pulses below the injury, and sensation to determine neurovascular status

    e. Elevate the limb to promote venous return and decrease edema

    f. Administer analgesics for pain relief

    g. Prepare the patient for surgery if an open reduction is necessary to stabilize the fracture

    h. Provide alternate means of mobility such as crutches or a wheelchair

    i. Instruct the patient to avoid weight bearing for 24 to 48 hours after experiencing a strain or sprain

    j. Teach the patient the importance of following instructions for activity limitation or exercise to restore limb function

G. Rape trauma
1. Introduction
    a. Rape is unlawful sexual intercourse without consent
    b. Rape is a legal term, not a medical diagnosis, and its definition may vary from state to state
    c. The involved parties may be men or women of any age
    d. The victim is usually female
    e. Rape itself is rarely a medical emergency unless rape-related trauma, such as stab wounds, lacerations, or fractures, exists
    f. Rape trauma represents a personal emergency for the victim and family
2. Assessment findings
    a. Severe emotional reaction
    b. Vaginal or rectal bleeding
    c. Vaginal, abdominal, or rectal pain
    d. Tachycardia
    e. Diaphoresis
    f. Semen and blood stains on the victim's clothing
    g. Bruises, cuts, or other injuries
3. Diagnostic test findings: constitute legal evidence
    a. Aspirated or scraped specimens from involved orifices: the male assailant's motile sperm and blood group antigen, and the presence of acid phosphatase in the semen
    b. Pubic hair scrapings: presence of the assailant's pubic hair
    c. Fingernail scrapings: presence of the assailant's skin and blood type
4. Patient care management goal: to provide emergency intervention with emotional support; to collect objective evidence if the victim wishes to prosecute; to administer prophylactic treatment for tetanus (if open wounds are present), infection, venereal disease, and pregnancy
    a. Keep in mind that the victim's informed consent is necessary for examination and treatment, as well as for the collection and the release of evidence to authorities
    b. Follow state law for collection of evidence and hospital protocol for the care of a rape victim
    c. Notify police, but recognize that the victim cannot be forced to talk to them
    d. Provide a person to remain with the victim at all times in a quiet, private, and nonthreatening environment
    e. Perform a thorough examination of the victim and treat any secondary complications
    f. Record a history of the incident as well as a sexual history, including birth control measures, date of last menstrual period, and pertinent medical history
    g. Make sure all specimen containers are properly labeled, include the initials of someone present during the examination, and are sealed with lids

h. Arrange for immediate patient counseling; put the patient in contact with a rape hot line counselor or rape crisis center
i. Treat open and contaminated wounds with tetanus prophylaxis and antibiotics
j. Provide protection against sexually transmitted diseases by administering penicillin and probenecid
k. Administer diethylstilbestrol to protect against pregnancy if the female victim is not using reliable contraception
l. Ensure that the victim has a family member or friend to stay with after hospital discharge
m. Provide all instructions and appointment information in writing so the victim will remember after the emotional crisis of rape
n. Make sure the victim understands the importance of medical follow-up to reevaluate the possibility of venereal disease and pregnancy

Points to Remember

Victims of trauma commonly have injury to more than one body system.

Narcotics prevent detection of changes in LOC and impair neurologic assessment.

Any chest injury is critical because chest injury is the leading cause of death for trauma victims.

Abdominal trauma may produce massive bleeding that is difficult to detect.

Examination and treatment of a rape victim as well as collection of evidence and its release to authorities require the victim's informed written consent.

Glossary

Concussion—injury caused by traumatic jarring of body tissue; common brain injury

Contusion—injury caused by traumatic bruising of body tissue; brain, chest, or abdomen injury

Flail chest—injury to the chest from a fracture of multiple ribs, a fracture of the ribs or sternum, or a fracture of three or more ribs in two or more places, creating a detached segment

Rhinorrhea—leakage of cerebrospinal fluid through the nose; commonly seen with a cranial fracture

Index

---

t refers to a table; i refers to an illustration.

t refers to a table; i refers to an illustration.

Notes

Notes

Notes

Notes

Notes

Notes

Notes

Notes

Notes